Louise Gibney grew up in Swindon but she currently lives in Milton Keynes. Her first novel on the perils of first dates promises cringing amusement and entertainment for all its readers.

Louise has had some poetry and short stories published in the past, but prefers to work on magazine articles and novels. She recommends to any budding writers that they join their local writers' group and advises them never to give up on their writing dreams.

Published in the UK
Copyright © Louise Gibney (2011)
Front cover design by Ciaran Robinson

9 781445 705569
ISBN 978-1-4457-0556-9
90000

'Girl Meets Boys'

Louise Gibney

GIRL MEETS BOYS

CONTENTS

The Checklist

Let me give you a quick summary of last year. Three of my friends (one of them my best friend) got married. My oldest girl friend from Primary School had her second (yep, second!) baby. The last of my university friends moved in with their other half. To top it all, my younger sister claimed that spinsterhood threatens everyone's door at least once in their life. It's alright for her – Tina and her man have been together for almost three years now. She didn't have to hammer that point home to me.

This is the time. This is when I should start my search for Mr Right. I'm new to Milton Keynes this summer and there should be some hope there alone in finding someone new.

So who am I? You know my name… I'm 24 years old, originally from Swindon, and I've spent some time living abroad in Canada. I thoroughly recommend doing so yourself if you have the chance – and not just for the expanded dating opportunities you'd find! I'm a mother to none, a friend to many. My family is larger than the average I'm told, but it just feels normal to me – I'm the eldest of three grown 'kids', trailed chronologically by Tina, an athletics obsessed blonde in a caring profession and Sam, my bright-spark brother who's training to be a pilot. I'm a curly haired brunette, a little on the petite (read short) side with a deceivingly un-dainty size 4.5 shoe. You'd think I'd have more grace when leaping up the stairs at home with feet that small, but no. My favourite footwear is flip flops or wellies (weather dependent of course) and I think a big reason why I enjoy camping so much is probably because there's virtually a guarantee that I get to wear both at some point in the trip!

I take pride in being pretty environmentally friendly, driving a small car, remembering my reusable shopping bags, and I recycle everything religiously. Part of it is sense, part of this is my green side poking through, but I also used to work in the recycling sector. I'm no hippy, I just think we, as temporary residents of this planet, should respect what natural beauties and variations we can see in the world and not spend their lives plundering their way through Earth's resources. Plus, why ruin it for future holiday escapes?! Now this sounds like a long-winded, preachy environmentalist's blog. I promise that's it for green-washing, dear reader.

I'm working on making writing more than a hobby, I enjoy travelling, watching movies and spending weekends by the sea. Oh yes, and I am single. Now this sounds like a Lonely Hearts column. Let's get on with the story.

I am single. I am not desperate, I assure you, but it just seems that all my friends are pairing up, moving in, having babies. And not just the serious stuff – couple's dinners, holidays with your man, 241 on Orange Wednesday cinema deals... I want to join in! I'm beginning a pursuit for romance, not a quest for something quick. See, I've always been a good girl, just ask my mum...

I don't make a habit of making boys my toys, but I know what I want and when I don't want it any more. *'How do I normally get what I want?'* I hear you ask. I write a list, that's how. So what do I want from a partner? Someone who intends on sticking around, will keep me on my toes, and will put up with my foibles for longer than a few months? What would I choose as ideal characteristics if I could magic a perfect man up from nowhere?

My Check List

Any future man of mine needs to...

1. Have a curious interest in the world – someone who enjoys travelling and current issues would fit the bill nicely
2. Be chatty but thoughtful
3. Enjoy his own interests (different to mine so we have something to keep each other occupied apart from the relationship)
4. Be family orientated – one day I'll want a family of my own
5. Hold at least half a brain inside his head. Braun is all very well, but on the other hand, I don't want to be scraping the barrel when it comes to intelligence!
6. Have a rugged Hugh Jackman look about him – my normal type seems to be anyone with a beard
7. Live close by. I'd like to be close enough to pop down for a quick cuppa (or something else...) if time is pressing one evening!
8. Be athletic to some degree

9. Enjoy watching films and listening to music – a common attribute, I'm sure, but we have to be able to enjoy films and music together without constant battles with the stereo/video rental card.
10. Wear a uniform to work. And I'm not talking B&Q uniform. Maybe this criteria is pushing my luck a little too far, but it *is* most girls' (including me) fantasy to have an affair with a fireman!

Phew, my list looks enormous now I've written it down! Is there a man out there who can tick half, let alone all of, my boxes?! It's like a 'To Do' list. Find a man with a good portion of these attributes and I'll have it made. The search starts today.

The Search Begins

So why am I so single? And what inspired me to write about my man hunt? I have had a splattering of relationships between school, university, moving to Canada and back to the UK again, in varied lengths of duration and involving a real variety of men. I figure I learnt something from every single one… that's what I keep telling myself anyway. One thing I did learn was that it's not so important to know what you want, more knowing what you *don't* want…

Having moved to an area which is unable to decide whether it's in the South East or the East Midlands, and not knowing anyone locally, the suggestion of internet dating was an intriguing idea to me. Since a couple of my friends had tried it with success before, I wondered what I had to lose. I thought, if nothing romantic came of it, I might at least make some new friends to help me settle into my new home town.

Who of you, dear readers, haven't had a cheeky look at online profiles? Tentatively at first, perhaps with a growing interest? According to a TV advert for a one dating website, 120,000 marriages result from online dating each year. I thought I'd give it a go – after all, people are proactive in every part of their lives, work, interests, so why not be proactive in moulding your love life? How else would you find such a wide range of single people ready to be contacted immediately? Relationships are one thing that makes life good or bad the majority of the time, so you'd be sensible to consider your full options in my opinion – one of those options being online dating – which is exactly why I logged on.

Online dating is starting to break through the barrier of embarrassment and taboo, and it's fast becoming a successful and celebrated way of meeting new people. The stigma has certainly lifted, and many shrewd business people are making a living out of exploiting single people's primal instinct to find a mate. Online dating has dismissed its reputation as being a matchmaker for the shy, weird and awkward, and has become much more acceptable and a juicy piece of gossip for all involved. Even the actress Halle Berry has allegedly had a glance around online.

Not wanting to blow my own trumpet…What does GSOH mean? What am I looking for? I'm new to the area – anyone up for showing me around? Just how *do* you start writing an online profile for yourself??? I'm a writer, shouldn't be too hard… I let my fingers ride my laptop's keys…

"Fun loving, independent, adventurous woman in her early 20's seeks hot and interesting entertainer to make her day, make her life."

Hmm. I scrapped shouting about being independent. It might scare the poor beggars off. 'Interesting'? That might open a whole other can of worms – there's no telling how 'interesting' this could get! And looking for an 'entertainer'? I definitely re-wrote this. I don't want to chance a kids' party clown showing up for a romantic evening in. Horrific idea, mainly because the squeak of balloons rubbing against each other makes my skin crawl. This short and mis-leadingly easy task of introducing myself to potential mates was proving harder than expected.

"A happy and confident brunette, I'm no high-maintenance handful. I love to laugh, watch films, and I bake a mean chocolate cake! I love spending time with family and friends and I enjoy traveling, seeing the world. Really looking for someone cute who can keep up with my adventures!"

Seven drafts later, this was an improvement, I think! Boy, that was hard work. Well, you know what they say, first impressions count for a lot, and I didn't want to rule too many out by being too sassy or in-your-face. Bulking out the intro with a couple of things I enjoy doing with my spare time definitely helped.

I then waded through the obligatory tick box exercise, filling in my name, age, location, height, profession, and your idea of a perfect first date. I said ice skating would hit the spot. I don't know why really – I have only skated once in my whole life when I was about eight years old. The whole afternoon consisted of me shuffling round the rink either clinging onto the barrier fence or sliding on my bum. Not an attractive view I imagine, but at least we'd have a laugh. And I'd never actually suggest that should a dating opportunity get that far down the line. Having second thoughts, I changed it to fruit picking. Weather dependent and seasonal, but at least you could get to know your date while picking (and eating!) your fruit, it's warmer than being on an ice rink, and you get some fresh air. Plus, I'm not aware of anyone who fruit picks spending the whole time sliding around on their arse or clinging to the fence in fear of their life. Perfect!

Text complete! Now, the daunting prospect of adding a photo. Something cute, but that's hard to achieve when the subject has an un-photogenic habit of closing your eyes in every shot. That's me! Finally finding a couple of acceptable photos, I bravely added them to the site. Three should do it. One of me dolled-up at a friend's wedding, (I scrub up well), one of me not looking my most sexy, but seemingly adventurous and able to look after myself, I hoped. This photo was taken near Cheddar Gorge with me admiring the landscape from a craggy rock, sporting a waterproof and a caving helmet. The final photo I chose was one I was looking relatively 'normal' in jeans and a tee, enjoying a cuppa at home. Vulnerable, warming. Hopefully *one* of those sides of me would appeal to someone browsing the site.

Online profile done. I did it! I logged off, enjoyed a long bath, daydreaming about the possibilities sure to come my way. I waited for the invites and emails to come flooding, or trickling, into my inbox.

A day in, and I'd already had some email interest, a couple of online 'winks', so obviously the photos weren't that horrific! However, they were no one who really appealed to me. As a writer and a keen reader, I know as well as any one shouldn't judge a book by its cover, or a man by the rugged angles of his cheek bones, but even the least judgemental have biases! Mine being dark hair, able show evidence of stubble growing capabilities, and someone taller than me. I cannot abide being limited to flat shoes (apart from my flip flops of course!) and I don't want to tower over my man – even at 5'4" it's possible, believe me.

I thought maybe I'd have a better chance of finding Mr Right if I found out something about someone from their online profile before I met them to try and spot if we had any common interests. The more you know about your ideal partner, the better your chances of winning them. I don't think online dating's just for weirdoes or losers if I'm one of the candidates registered on there under the world's scrutiny – I think I am normal enough.

An Australian friend of mine moved to Canada shortly after we studied together at Ontario's Brock University. He met a lovely Canadian girl through a dating website. They moved in together after a few months. Now happily married, they were definitely a catalyst to me signing up online. Really, I could try to blame what follows all on them... Thanks guys! Since then, another of my school friends has married an online date, and they have two little girls now, so there's something in the proof of *that* pudding, that's for sure.

Some people still have a fear or shyness about going online. Most people would rather find themselves locked out in the buff than sign up, but I was brave enough to try it out. My attitude is, have no fear, no embarrassment – you're in the same boat as each other. There's a possibility of momentary awkwardness on the first date, or some embarrassment on admitting the details of how you met to other people if it works out, but it'll be worth it if you find The One.

Of course, there are certain sensible rules I made for myself, which, unfortunately from the horror stories you can find, I doubt everyone seems to use to protect themselves well enough. It's worth noting I always made sure I was dating safely, never meeting anyone anywhere I felt uncomfortable, always telling someone where I was and when I expected to be back. After all, you don't know who these people are, as much as you may have talked to them on the phone or on IM (Instant Messaging) before meeting them – unfortunately there's way too many liars and perverts in this world. I'm a sensible girl me.

Some general points (to reassure you I haven't lost my mind)

- I never told any first dates where I lived. No one needs a nutty stalker.
- While sifting through potential online dates, stay in control. Browse the pool on offer before signing up, and don't let some guy from the website's headquarters office in Milwaukee decide who your soul mate is. Matching people's personalities doesn't always work out – I for one wouldn't like to date my double.
- Also, make sure you can specify your no-no's – my friend Jenn, who we'll meet later, is often frustrated when websites don't let you put a limit on how short a date can be. This can be an obstacle if you're a tall beauty like Jenn.
- Give them a chance – just because you don't want to jump their bones the second your eyes meet doesn't mean you won't have a fantastic evening out anyway
- I never got picked up from home, or told anyone where I

worked, keeping details kinda vague. It amazes me when I hear stories of people telling complete strangers where they live, all about the pubs they're "always in, every night", and where their kids go to school

- I don't have any kids, but rule number one for any mothers - posting how old their children are along with pictures on your profile page? Perfect information for a paedophile stalker, I'd imagine.
- And lastly, join with a friend. Moral support is exactly that – a friendly boost based on personal conviction or experience – and everyone should have someone they can divulge all their date stories filled with cringes, intrigue and laughs.

My friend Rachel was occasionally on-call to phone me after a quick emergency text message from me saying "call me in ten mins" so I could make up some 'urgent' getaway if needs be – a brilliant exit strategy. It was normally "a mate's car's just broken down and she's stranded" or "our boiler's just exploded" or something ridiculous like that.

Well, at the end of the day, I thought I'd give it a go. Gone are the days of Tea Dances and the Feudal System ranking everyone into planned relationships (good and bad), and I was sick of meeting people in nightclubs the modern 'traditional' way. It really wasn't getting me anywhere, with or without naff chat up lines. I might be heavily stereotyping here, as I for one am not like this, but a lot of people I have met out on the town are only after one thing: a quick fix to a lonely evening. You must have seen or heard the classic, romantic line at the end of the night when a glassy eyed Romeo broaches the suggestion of leaving together with "You'll do..."

I have met the exception to the rule, but not many people engage in a fling which started in a bar and make it last longer than one night. Bars are deceiving – people arrive in groups, tend not to mingle, and then also leave in a group. You could be introduced to someone via friend, but even that can be a minefield.

I set about sifting through potential dates online, admittedly with a strong bias towards dark haired, masculine types, often with a five o'clock shadow or more, and with a good grasp of the English language. There's nothing wrong with not wanting someone who doesn't know how to use a spell checker (case in point, Chinese Charlie). For goodness sake, you're on the computer already, why not run your profile text by Mr Spell Check before clicking on that all too revealing 'publish' button?

A negative attitude, stilted and limited conversation, and people who contact you in the first instance with a line like "you're fit, wanna chat?" is such a turn-off. If something doesn't feel right, it's probably not. You have to learn how to sift through the weirdoes and the liars.

I also don't like it when men start their emails with something like "hey babe, wanna chat?" That tells me nothing about them, or why they're interested in chatting, so you have to assume they're after one thing. Lonely internet sex. I like to see a personalised email so it shows they've picked you out especially to email, and are actually interested in who you are. One-liners may work when speaking to someone face-to-face, but not on email. It's more than likely to be spam.

One more thing – unless I'm really intrigued or especially tempted, I won't contact a guy who just has the minimum information on his online profile. Some cases just put a picture up and put the obligatory details of age, sex, location. These guys are just not taking this seriously enough in my opinion.

This book is a collection of true stories where girl (me) meets boys (them) in an attempt to find that something more. Whether it's a date found online or a more normal liaison, every word written here was a true occurrence – I'm far too honest to make anything up. All names and most places (where not implicit to the story) have been changed to protect the identity of the nice and the not so nice…This is Girl Meets Boys.

A Curious Interest in the World

I should have listened to my mother!

It doesn't matter who you talk to, most girls have had a man who turned their life inside out. Even for a short period of time. He probably doesn't even realise he's doing it, making us feel used but still head-over-heels. He can leave a girl miserable, confused, and despondent about men in general, yet we still retain more than a healthy interest. Arben was such a man.

Arben was the waiter for our table at my friend's leaving dinner do, and it was clear to my mates that something was sparking between us. However, maternal instincts and advice, I reluctantly admit, are right the majority of the time. Had my mother been there, she would have chastised me carefully and made me feel guilty for even window shopping. Maybe I should have heeded my mum's gentle, albeit deemed slightly racist and out-dated warning about foreign waiters when I met Arben.

However. This guy was gorgeous! If only I had a photo to share with you, but as you can imagine from the nature of this book, we never got that far into the relationship for me to start snapping photos. What kind of keen freak takes a camera on the first couple of dates?! Not me! Anyway, Arben was, and still is, tall, with dark features, dark hair just short enough, and broad built. All winners in my book, but the foreign twang in his accent made him even more appealing. What is it about accents, people either love them or hate them? We ended up swapping phone numbers and he texted me later that evening to arrange to go out for drinks. Everything seems like a good idea until afterwards…

We had a lovely evening out in an upmarket bar in Milton Keynes. It turns out Arben's cousin got him a job in the restaurant a couple of months ago, after moving to the UK from Albania. He was fun, intelligent, and mysterious, and Arben wasn't shy about his feelings towards me from the outset. It was nice to go out with someone with a bit of 'get up and go', someone with an apparent lust for travelling and adventure to match mine. I fell, hook, line and sinker. Or should it be 'stinker'? This did not have a happy ending, you can probably guess.

Albanian Arben was enthusiastic about travelling, much like I am, and promised to be my personal tour guide if I ever fancied visiting his home nation of Slovenia and the rest of Eastern Europe. Yes, Slovenia, you didn't read it wrong. I didn't notice at the time that he was so vague about where he originated from (I admit, the level of knowledge I have about East European geography is ignorant at best). Slovenia, Albania… He kept changing his mind. It should have been my first sign.

Our second date was squeezed in right before I flew out to New Zealand for a fortnight. Arben took me out to dinner at Nando's – his favourite restaurant. I'm not sure why he liked it so much. It's pretty much fast food in a canteen in my view, so I'm not too fussed by it. It was a fun evening anyway, so I can't judge it too badly. And have since gone back! Well, maybe it's not just my standards of men which have potentially slipped…

On the way back to the car Arben made me promise I'd come back for him after my trip, and in return he promised to collect me from the airport. I was told in no uncertain but mildly jokey terms that I'd have to 'behave' while I was having fun the other side of the world, but he said he would be looking forward to seeing me again. Slightly concerned by Arben's keen interest in me and the light-hearted instructions on not playing deviant while on holiday, (after all, this was still only our second date, and surprisingly, I'm not attracted to stalkers), I gave him a cheesy wink and said I'd be back. I wasn't going to let him know he was definitely in for a third date. Something to look forward to after coming down to Earth with a bump on my return I hoped.

I had a fantastic couple of weeks away, bombing around the New Zealand countryside in a hire car, sucking in all the scenery, caving, ice hiking, partying and meeting lots of people. I could go on, but this is not a travel blog.

Arben emailed me a couple of times while I was away, always ending with a comment about how he was looking forward to meeting me at Heathrow. I couldn't wait to have someone in Arrivals waiting for me – I am always insanely jealous when I see other travellers being met by friends and family, getting hugs, flowers, balloons and smiles.

My return flight to London was perfect. The flight itself was great, and my dad, who works for the airline, surprised me by appearing on the flight with a welcome home card from my mum, dad, and grandparents. I think they were worried I wouldn't come home after such a fab time away. Tempting – New Zealand is such a fantastic place! This was a brilliant surprise and I spilled (almost) all of my adventures to Dad for a good couple of hours while we flew back to Blighty.

I was so excited to see Dad – then it dawned on me… Arben was picking me up in Arrivals. Dad knew nothing about this new man on the scene. We'd only been on two dates, so I wasn't quite ready for the whole 'meet the parents' situation which was fast unravelling before my eyes. As an unforgiving bonus, my dad has a not-so secret dislike towards Albanians, and had warned me off them for some reason several years ago. This exciting and romantic reunion of mine and Arben's was turning out to be a nightmare. Not at all how I'd planned!

I decided to come clean to my dad about my anticipation of being met by a romantic liaison of mine at Arrivals, and I pleaded with him to let me walk through alone ahead of him to warn my unsuspecting date that my dad would be following shortly. It was only fair, the poor bloke.

However, Arben wasn't there. I stood in Arrivals at Heathrow Airport confused, disappointed, and a little mad, wondering where the hell he was. I'd gone through all the grief of explaining it to my dad as well. The cheek of it.

Dad soon followed me through Arrivals and saw me standing on my own. I explained that Arben wasn't there and his phone was turned off. I sent him a text asking where he was, and I'd get the National Express home if he wasn't here within half an hour. My father obviously wasn't impressed with this at all. And this was without him knowing he was Albanian! Half an hour passed. Still no show. Dad and I went home. Dad was probably a little relieved that this automatically assumed moron hadn't shown up, but I drove home with my tail firmly between my legs. Awkward in the driver's seat, but you get the idea!

Two days later Arben's phone was still turned off. I blame what follows on my jet lag. Partly out of concern and partly consumed by some of the curiosity that killed the cat, I called Arben's restaurant to find out what had happened. Apparently he'd been arrested and demoted at work as he'd missed a shift, being locked up and all. I'd pretty much written off him as a potential boyfriend at this point.

Arben called me three days later. His explanation for leaving me stranded at Heathrow Airport was that he'd gone to pick me up in his old banger of a car and got caught speeding. He didn't have a valid MOT or tax disc so the police locked him up for the night. Consequently he missed my arrival back to London. To this day I still don't know how truthful this story was…

Anyway, he begged me unapologetically to give him another chance. I swear, dear reader, that these were his exact words: "come on *mate*, give me another chance" – what's he doing calling me 'mate'? This is where I should have said no. No, no, no!

Of course, we went out for drinks again, and things looked more promising, even though I'd still not got an apology for the unceremonious ditching I got on return from my holiday. He dropped me home and went home himself.

The next day I saw he'd changed his Facebook status from 'single' to read 'in an open relationship'. WHAT? That ain't my cuppa tea, sunshine. I phoned Arben and we had a mini domestic about an open relationship *not* being what I wanted, and him insisting repeatedly that it was a joke. Ha. Ha. Did he actually want me to agree to that? What would my friends think? The guy I'm dating is open to other women? Anyway, I made him change his status changed back to single – the preferred option to that 'open relationship' rubbish.

Arben called me the following day after our 'words' to say our plans to go to dinner in a couple of days had to be put on hold. Could I please come round, bringing a Chinese takeaway, and look after him as he'd broken his ankle. Whatever next? He'd injured himself kicking someone to a pulp because they'd taken his parking space the night before. Wonderful. Brilliant news.

My naïve sympathy is easy to acquire though, so I dutifully went to the newsagents for his crisp and cigarette supplies, (dirty habit, what was I thinking?) and got the Chinese in. I loaned Arben some DVDs to keep him occupied, after his pathetic puppy looks and moaning that he couldn't "focus on being lovely to me" while he was in this state. Hmm…

A few days later he lost his job due to his incapacity to work. It was a hard story to drag out from his lips, but as he was an illegal immigrant (!) he had no entitlement to sick pay. This meant he had to move out of his flat and live with his cousin, almost two hours away until his foot improved. Two hours away. No way was I going to travel that far and back home for an evening with such a troublesome date. He didn't even offer me to stay over as he knew I'd probably not want to stay in a three bedroom squat with seven other men. What a perceptive bloke. Best off out of that one – his 'world interest' wasn't for travelling, but scamming illegal entry into better countries than his own.

OK Cupid, at that point it became the long-overdue end for me. He did say maybe we could pick up where we left off later in the year when his ankle had healed, but I knew that wasn't going to happen. He sent me an email in January asking "if I was still mad" – I was never mad. In disbelief of the circumstances, yes, but not mad. I gave him a friendly "piss off" and told him not to contact me anymore. Arben may have had a 'curious interest in the world', as preferred by me, but I wasn't after illegal immigrants who fancied their chances somewhere better off.

BlueAndWhite

23 years old

6'2'', athletic build

Milton Keynes – new to town!

Describe yourself…

I'm originally from Greece, into movies and going to gigs, and I have a good sense of humour – I think! My friends would say I am a friendly, loyal type, who never gives up – in a non-creepy way lol!

What are you looking for?

Someone to show me around Milton Keynes – there's got to be a lot of first date opportunities in this city!

Normal and Decent

What I liked about Alexis initially was that he made a real effort with his emails. Emails are great for screening people – if you read them carefully you can tell if the writer is typing how they'd normally speak. They also make good tools for comparisons between different people. I've known other girls to even print off emails from men and file them, showing friends the details to see if they approve. Anyway, Alexis seemed nice, he had plenty of (good looking) pictures to prove it was actually him I was speaking to. Plus, he was Greek – something different for me and he seemed interested in exploring the world (and Milton Keynes!). His accent must be divine!

We decided that as he was relatively new to town, (newer than me, only having moved there a month ago), I should show him around his new patch. This plan, I hoped brought lots of opportunity to talk on a nice sunny summer's afternoon, and we could build in dinner, drinks, sightseeing – whatever we fancied.

So my and Alexis' date rolled around, and thus begun another semi-mundane mating ritual as I showed him around some of the delights that Milton Keynes has to offer. Picnickers enjoying the sun sitting by the concrete cows, the ski dome, cable boarding at Willen Lakes, a whistle-stop tour of the theatre district…I'd rather be *doing* some of these things, but watching was fine for now. I was secretly making mental notes of future date ideas, with or without Alexis.

We dined at a local seafood restaurant for dinner, which made a nice change. As much as Alexis loved seafood (well, he is Greek after all!), I didn't think dinner was a good time to mention a bit of trivia I know about the mating rituals of the critters on our plates. A romantic seafood dinner might have quickly become unappetising had I mentioned that lobsters urinate during foreplay or that male octopi get it on with a specially designed 'baby making' arm!

A film followed dinner - 'In Bruges', the Colin Farrell action movie. The movie was good, and Alexis was a lovely guy, but more action happened in those 107 minutes of film than our three hours of dating. Sure, he'd travelled the world and had the guts to up sticks and live abroad, but unfortunately, we had scored a zero score on the spark-o-meter. He was a nice enough guy, but there's a lot to be said for that elusive spark. You know the kind – the one that makes you feel an actual flutter in your stomach. It makes your palms feel sweaty even if they're not. You wonder if you've read the signs wrong and worry he's not feeling the same. You can't wait for another 'accidental' brush of your arms as you walk through another the door he holds open. Your mind goes into overdrive full of emotion and plans should this all work out. I'm getting full of romantic tension just writing about it! Maybe I should try erotica for my next novel. Erm, yes, back to Alexis.

So the spark wasn't there, and really, he was a little shy too. Sure, he was gentlemanly, but a little bland. Polite but rude in appropriate occasions is preferred to the 'good boy well-behaved' option. Although we had spent a pleasant afternoon, we didn't stay in touch. We left it as "if you want to hang out, help finding your feet in town, you know here I am" but it fizzled to nothing rapidly – maybe he was hoping for more than just a tour guide. I'm not even sure if he's still in the UK. It was a lovely way to spend an afternoon though, nice to meet someone new and normal. It does prove however that 'the spark' is not a myth and you really can't fake it as much as you might want to. Maybe he didn't like British girls? Had I ruined his high hopes of finding an English Rose? Because I'm certainly not that – remember my not-so-dainty size 4.5 feet, tanned skin and dark Hispanic-esque hair, and complete lack of endearing freckles perhaps more akin to the stereotyped English appearance? To be honest, I looked more classically Greek than Alexis, with his mousey hair and un-Godlike confidence!

Perhaps I should re-address my 'must-have' personality trait of any potential date having a curious interest in the world. Maybe a clause about being British to start with? Judging by Alexis and Arben both unsuccessfully stumbling through their dates, it might root out the travellers and adventurers in Milton Keynes, rather than the migrants.

Computer Says No

Just one internet date in (Alexis - remember, Arben the immigrant was a waiter I just came across), and my laptop decided to give up the ghost. Should I have taken this as a sign?!

Now, I'm no computer genius, but when a black screen appears with white script scrolling in front of my eyes I know *something's* up. How frustrating – not only was this probably going to cost me a bomb to fix, it meant I'll be offline and away from the online dating scene for a few days or weeks. I hadn't realised how addicted to casually browsing the fields of faces posted online I'd become! I'd barely scratched the surface! Nowadays I'd just use my smart phone to feed my addiction while the computer was being looked at, but I didn't have one back then.

So, at the first opportunity I had, I took my computer into my local electronics repair shop. It had been recommended by a colleague who'd had similar problems with his laptop last month. They were surely to be trusted to look after my laptop, my key to the online dating world.

I breezed into the shop, a little worried with a fringe of doubt that my poor computer could ever be saved. There were no other customers in the shop, and the guy behind the shop's counter stood with his back to me. He heard me lump the laptop carrying case onto the front desk of the shop and turned to greet me.

Wow, nice tan. That wasn't out of a bottle, but didn't go well with the blue and orange uniform he was probably a little embarrassed to be seen in (I hoped!). I briefly wondered where he'd travelled to get such a deep matt complexion mid-November before he welcomed me with a smile. "How can I help?"

Ah, customer service with a smile - I liked that. Right, I had his full attention and began to pour my laptop woes at his feet. Why is it that whenever I have to explain a technical fault in something, be it my laptop, my car, or my phone, I start rambling and start including inconsequential things.

"Well, I just went off to get a fresh cuppa and when I returned…"

Or "It was just the last thing I needed after I'd also broken my oven doorknob off the same morning".

My words run away with themselves and I end up sounding like an ignorant technophobe. Oh, ok, you got me, I kind of am. I love my gadgets but only when they're working!

Max (staff name badges, invaluable source of information!) chatted away, reassuring me he'd have a good look at my laptop. Satisfied that Max would have it ready for me in a couple of days, I turned to leave the shop, thanking the helpful technician.

"Wait," I heard. "I see you have a Maple Leaf's Ice Hockey key chain."

Jangling my keys suggestively towards him, I now realise (oops, reign it in girl!), I twirled round. No one in the UK knows who The Leafs are!

"What affiliation do you have with Canada? I'm off that way myself this summer – any tips?" he enquired.

A keen traveller obviously. I gave Max a quick brief on what to do and where to avoid. Always willing to share some of the locals' tips I'd learned living near The Falls in Niagara, I wished him a safe trip. I felt like my precious date-finding laptop was in safe hands.

*   *   *

Returning home that evening, my housemate Tom promised to help calm my online dating cold turkey. Over the next couple of days or so while I waited for helpful Max to fix my own laptop, I could continue my search online on Tom's PC for a man perfect enough for me.

Chatty, But Thoughtful

FriendlyMKbloke

27 years old

5'9" tall, slim build

Milton Keynes

Describe yourself…

A is for … adventurous

B is for … basketball fan

C is for … chatty camper who can't stand caravans

D is for … dark haired, but light hearted

E is for … Well, I shouldn't spoil all my mystery straight away!!

What are you looking for?

Someone local who can make me smile. I'm looking for that "spark" as I think there's no point just being in a relationship for the sake of it.

Jail Bird Blues

Adventurous, dark, tall, friendly. He even mentioned camping in his online CV – sorry, profile. Fabien looked great on paper. He was also a successful IT consultant. Geek, you think? Well, sources tell me geek is the new cool, and judging by the popularity of shows like 'Glee' and 'The Inbetweeners', I think they might be right. And a proven technophobe like me knows any help is welcome when you need help installing a new printer or defragging your computer.

Fabien and I chatted online regularly like old friends for about a month (chatty – check!), before we planned a lunch date at our local Wetherspoons bar. Not very imaginative, I know. A huge amount of dating success in a bar location depends on what type of establishment you decide to meet in – snug and cosy with a roaring fire? Happy Hour in the trendy vodka bar? - but they do good burgers at 'Spoons. Pubs are also a good option to arrange a 'coincidental' meeting with your friends. A conveniently well-timed second opinion anyone? Plus, the drinks are cheap if he's tight-fisted.

Anyway, Fabien's big day quickly was upon us. That afternoon when I'd finished work and was heading into town to meet him, I wondered if that was the hint of a butterfly flutter in my stomach. Or it could be the questionable curry I'd had before rearing its ugly Masala head. I hoped and was pretty sure it was the former rather than the latter. I was really looking forward to meeting Fabien. Note to self – no curries even the night before meeting a potential mate.

However, it all came to an end before it started. I found myself ditched at the bar. I didn't have a number to call him on (I *so* need to get over the fear of stalkers and swap phone numbers more), so I went home a little disgruntled. Where was he?!

Fabien emailed me the next day to explain that he had a 'family issue' to deal with that day. I was highly sceptical, as it's such a convenient 'get out' excuse. I had no idea at the time even if he *had* a family to speak of at this point, but I took it as an honest story. Little did I know, but all was forgiven far too soon. It turns out this honest lad wasn't so honest. Anyway, Fabien was given the benefit of the doubt when he assured me he was keen to set a date for another drink some time. That's using your initiative and shows you're serious, boys.

Date two (lucky guy it seems to get a second date, judging by how many chapters we have left here!) was a drink in my village pub. I'm no expert on body language, but I think the feeling of attraction was mutual, as I noticed I found I was subconsciously mirroring his pose.

Bring out the body language!

Parted lips mean sexual desire is bubbling inside, but was he just gasping for a beer?

I've heard of people **fiddling with their clothes** being a sure sign they're interested, perhaps imagining slowly peeling your clothes off, or over-run with nerves… or maybe he's got a wedgie?

Fiddling with anything (ahem!) seems to be a good sign in general in fact. If a guy is playing with the empty glass in front of him, you're most probably still in the game. However, he may just be wondering when you were going to get the next round in.

Folded arms, a defensive pose – not on our table that night!

Someone who's **twirling locks of their hair in their fingers** is a very unscientific way of guessing they're interested in you, too. Or, maybe that new shampoo smell rubbing off on their fingers is an irresistible distraction.

Stroking their face/chin/neck, and **raising an eyebrow** – this definitely means he's interested, unless of course he's fresh from a round of Botox.

We were **both leaning in towards each other** when speaking (and not because I'm deaf!). Definitely a good sign!

Fabien was very complimentary towards me all evening, saying he expected me to be a hippy as I was in my environmentally friendly phase. In fact, he said I was "very easy on the eyes". A back-handed compliment. Wow, he's a keeper…

Sarcasm aside, whether I was receiving good or bad body language signals, (and obviously they're open to much criticism, I'm no psychologist), I couldn't get a word in edgeways all evening. Camping was an obvious starter for icebreaking, but we talked about all manner of things. Travel plans, ideal jobs, phone contracts, the pain of driving tests… Chatty as he was, it was secretly quite funny how much and how fast Fabien spoke. I assumed it was just nerves, until it clicked. He talked a lot about his "past involved in drugs", and I have a strong feeling that Fabien was on speed (or something similar – I'm no expert!) that night. Not good. Anyway, it was an enjoyable evening, but on the way out of the pub, Fabien lit up a cigarette (he had said he'd quit) and, sin of mortal sins, he dropped the empty packet on the ground. Eurgh, don't be a tosser – take your litter home with you!

On Monday morning, after hearing my account of my date with Fabien, colleagues at work recommended at this point I don't go in for a third date, perhaps me mixing with company where drug use is commonplace being their primary concerns.

So, why did I give Fabien a third date? He said he owed me a steak dinner for stitching me up for lunch that time and I found it hard to turn down, even with the previous doubts I had. He was gorgeous, and I love steak. Date number three was even more enlightening about our dear Fabien…

- He rang me beforehand to ask what clothes I'd like him to wear – dress yourself, man!

- He'd lost his driving license for one reason or another so I was his taxi driver for all and any dates we might decide to go on

- He told me he'd been arrested three times in two years for various street trading crimes

- He was open about how he frequently scams money on various projects and commits minor naughties in local shops. This included a tax avoidance admission – who would tell a tax-payer they're conniving to get out of the monthly HM Rev & Customs salary deduction and expect a warm and respectful response?!

- He talked about drug use A LOT. I feared this was more than a 'former' past-time…

- He flashed his money about when the bill came. He took what appeared to be more that £100 out for a pub meal with me. I don't like show-offs. Money doesn't maketh the man – manners do!

Not cool. I told Fabien I'd rather just be friends (although I'd really rather not) and contact between us ended abruptly. Let's just say he's not someone I'd like to bring home to show my parents. They'd get sick of the sound of his voice no doubt. I've seen it before – they don't like chatty boyfriends dating their daughters, especially ones suspected of drug use. As for me, yes, chatty is on my list of preferences in a man, but not at the expense of his health, my drug-free life, and the rocky future liaisons with such a crowd could bring. Call me chicken, call me square, but I've never had any involvement in recreational drugs and I prefer it that way. End of.

BeatlesFan222

31 years old

5'7" tall, average build

Banbury

Describe yourself…

I'm Lewis, from Banbury, and I'm a huge Beatles fan. I am interested in meeting new people from around the area. I like music, films, and the outdoors. I've been single about a year and thought I'd try something different by coming on here. Here's hoping!

What are you looking for?

Someone I'll look forward to spending my free time with - no "crazies" please!

A Pig Awful Date

Lewis was the next in a long line of serial one-date-only male prospects. We'd chatted on the phone a couple of times in addition to emailing through the match making website. This was something way off the beaten date track for me, as I'm very protective of my phone number and hardly ever give it out. The hassle of spam texts, perhaps having to change my number or blocking someone else's from my phone is something I'd rather not be burdened with. Lewis's internet was disconnected the last week of his dating website membership though due to a house move, so

I thought, despite the Beatle's fan poor and out-dated taste in music, what the hell, jump in, let's meet up.

The Tuesday we chose to rendez-vous on was a wet and windy night, so I suggested we take shelter in a Mexican restaurant I'd been eyeing up. It was middle-of-the-road kind of place, not too expensive, not too scummy, but it also turned out to be one of the first casualties of the 'credit crunch'. It had closed down the previous week. Bugger. Added to that disappointment, Lewis was also a lot older than his online photos lead me to think - double bugger. Anyway, I thought 'oh well', I was already there, I'd committed, and I was starving. So, in the absence of Mexican munch, we went next door to a pleasant looking Italian place. I'm all about trying international food, me!

In all honesty, this Tuesday was probably bad timing for a date, probably with any unlucky candidate. It followed a rocky weekend with a long-term fling (who'd decided to dump me preferring one of my best friend's sisters), so I might not have been in the best frame of mind… However, I believe that love can be a bit like basketball. When a ball sails hopefully towards the hoop to score, sometimes it bounces off the hoop or the back board to return to play. I used to enjoy having the important job of keeping score for a basketball team an ex too boring to chapter in this book played for. Watching the training sessions and scoring the matches, a rebound occurred to me as simply something that will put you back in the game. Harry Potter fans unite, you're forbidden to speak the guy's name from this weekend's hurtful slam dunk dumping out loud. My family have named him 'Voldermort'. Voldermort's exit to my life meant I needed a fast recovery. A rapid rebound. Sitting in that Italian, avoiding the eyes of any waiters (remember Arben?), I was hoping the basketball metaphor was an appropriate one for Lewis.

Rebound material or not, my date with Lewis had already started badly with two disappointing events (his photo obviously taken about 10 years ago, and the closed down restaurant). Are you ready for the next one?

Get this – Lewis's favourite topic of conversation was pig breeding. No joke! Where to stage the mating session, how to get the best stock, what to do with the 'retirees', the (ahem) size of the studs… Oh boy. He wasn't even a pig farmer for a living. Pig farming was eight years ago. He's now a builder. Thank goodness I had chosen a delicious lamb dinner over pork chops that evening.

Our long-winded and sometimes stomach churning conversation ended after about half an hour. It had been a mainly one-way discussion, surprisingly enough, considering the topic, and now moved onto slightly less boring subjects like how much beer he drinks and DIY projects. I do drink at least, not as much as Lewis, but I can at least relate in some way to that (unlike pig farming). And DIY – I do have a hammer at home, somewhere…

Chatty Lewis made a move to redeem himself marginally when he walked me back to my car and asked if he could show me his pick up truck.

'*OK, nice*' I thought, I love a man with a pick up.

This one was NOT what I was hoping for though. It stank, and looked like it had just come in from throwing pig swill out on the fields, a right old banger. I was wishing on a shiny new Dodge Ram or a Mitsubishi Warrior. Granted, it *was* the real McCoy here, put to good use at a building site or hog studding field somewhere, but there's nothing sexy about that.

So, that was Pig Farmer Lewis. We had a nice dinner, but it wasn't going to progress any further than that. Am I too picky? Hmmm, I think not. His conversation, chatty as it was, was not my cup of tea. Standing in the multi-storey car park, freezing my arse off in the cold wind, I made some lame excuse up about having to pick up my friend from the station at 8.30pm. So, "unfortunately" I said faking an appropriately remorseful expression, we didn't have time for after dinner drinks.

That being said, after my sharing of the story of Pig Farmer Lewis, my friend Jenn came up with the wise words of "Bad dates are OK". After all, we singletons are not learning the hard way, it's the fun way! Jenn's convinced the more awful dates you have the more you know what you want from a man. Err… Has she seen my track record?! Perhaps a tick list of qualities is the wrong way to go about my mission. Maybe a list of "no thanks!" characteristics would be more useful!

You Never Know Where You Might Pick Up!

Let me take you back a year or two. I *was* dating before I got a laptop, of course! Before I lived in Milton Keynes, I spent a period of time living in Northampton due to securing a new job in the area. I was living in a town house shared by six professionals with various nationalities ranging from Spanish and French to Japanese. I was settling in nicely, but as it was a pretty multicultural house with different shift patterns, no one really spent any time together. Not ideal when I knew no one in Northampton. So, bored, I decided I would have to invest in a TV for my room.

Not the most exciting past-time, but at least the evenings I was spending in the house would pass a little quicker, programmes at a volume to distract me from the what seemed like constant humping noises coming from upstairs and the wailing of my neighbour singing along to her Will Young CDs.

I'd found a great store in the town run by the British Heart Foundation, where people can donate household goods to the charity and the shop sells them on for profit. I thought my luck was guaranteed there for success in finding a cheap, reliable TV. In more ways than I expected, it turns out.

One Saturday morning, I perused the electronics section, glancing about pretending I knew more about TVs than I actually did. This was before the days of 3D and HD, but I still felt bamboozled by the choice of electronics available, even in this charity store. Black, blue, silver and grey in colour - even pink was in stock. And how can I possibly be expected to estimate the screen size? Don't the manufacturers know we measure in centimetres now, not inches? Did I want a remote? Not bothered, I guessed. My rented room wasn't big enough to not get up off my butt to change the channel.

A helpful, handsome member of staff spotted my obvious confusion and he came over to help. Jake, his name tag suggested I call him. I couldn't help noticing he was tall, dark, and had a wide perfectly toothed smile. He was probably more flirty than helpful, but he eventually got a sale when I settled on a heavy duty black TV set. What can I say? Jake had amazing sales schmoozing performance skills!

Having picked out a suitable 'tube', I willingly followed his broad shoulders to the till station to pay. As Jake filled out the TV license request form for me, he asked me for my phone number. I thought, well, if he's in any way inclined to be a stalker he'd get it off my TV license form anyway. He was cute, so I thought why not.

I think Jake exceeded the 'service with a smile' sales technique. You know the type. Customer orientated and more than helpful. I'd go back to that store any day! He helpfully carried the TV out to my car and continued the blatant flirt tactics and said "maybe I'll call you around 7pm tonight"… Maybe I'd be in!

When he did call, Jake and I chatted for a while and he asked me out on a date. I was more than happy at this proposition, but we couldn't decide on something to do. Apparently, he didn't like going out for meals, films bored him, pubs and clubs weren't his cup of tea, and he said it was not the right kind of weather for relaxing in a park etc. – all of which I fail to believe as it was late summer, and who doesn't enjoy going for drinks and a meal somewhere?

Well, I decided I'd leave the ball in his court, especially since I was heading out in a few minutes to have dinner with a friend, so we ended the call. He was assigned the responsibility of choosing a suitable date for us at the weekend.

The next day Jake rang me back with the news he couldn't think of anything for a date. How convenient and imaginative! He suggested he came over to the house and we could 'chill' at mine. Not ideal by far. I had no idea who he was, didn't really want him to know where I lived, and especially to see the noisy, cosmopolitan house I lived in with a bunch of people who never cleaned up and barely spoke English. I knew exactly what he was planning in his little man brain. Booty call! I politely declined. I wonder how many other British Heart Foundation customers he'd got numbers from…

Jake obviously got the message I wasn't going to jump into anything fast, his bed in particular, and he never called me again. Well, I never thought buying a TV might (almost) get me a date. He was certainly ticking the 'chatty' box, but perhaps was not hitting the right 'thoughtful' notes… Oh, and I still have the TV. Second (could be third) hand and mine for over five years, still going strong.

Ice_Hockey_Josh

30 years old

5'11" tall, average build

Milton Keynes

Describe yourself…

I like listening to music (Blur, Oasis, Kasabian, The Killers etc) and my new year's resolution this year was to see more live acts. I'm doing quite well, one every month so far! I'm into horror films, but don't worry, I don't bite!

What are you looking for?

Open to all types – I don't believe people only have one type they go for every time. Who's to say something new isn't the answer to your search?

Boring Banker Alert!

Banker (careful…!) Josh, almost breaking the 30 years boundary, was one of my older dates. We established after chatting for a while, that we both enjoyed watching ice hockey. Both also having meant to go to the local games more often, we thought what better place to meet than the arena to get to know each other. There was ample opportunity to get to know each other too, refreshments available, and the entertainment of the match to sit and watch quietly should the conversation dried up. A great date idea really.

Match day, we chatted in the stands and got to know each other a little, but again, like Pig Farmer Lewis, Josh was nothing like his photo. He had put on a significant amount of weight since then. Note of caution: Approach 'average build' with caution - what one person thinks is average may not be your idea of average. Love may be blind but dating, online or otherwise, generally isn't.

While we're on the subject of photos, it still surprises me the number of people whose main online photo, the one you'd see first from their profile on a search, is of them in fancy dress. Sure, the subject looks fun-loving maybe, and might suggest you wouldn't say no to a party (or other things involving costumes) but at least show your face. Hiding under woolly hats and sunglasses is another no-no. Another thing I also give people a wide berth for is when their photo is taken with their arm up in the air at a weird angle. It's obvious it's been taken by themselves with their mobile phone. Have they no friends help photograph them?

Anyway, back to Josh. He kindly shouted me a hot chocolate, ticking the 'thoughtful and friendly' box, but Josh's conversation on all things related to finance really didn't excite me. Why do so many blokes only talk about their work? It could be because such men have nothing else in their life, which doesn't bode well for the 'have his own interests' criteria.

On the drive home, it occurred to me that the only downside to choosing the ice hockey match for our date's venue was the chance of having the awkward situation arise of bumping into my former and unsuccessful date at a game again later on in the hockey season. I've been along since a couple of times, but luckily that ticking time bomb has yet to explode. Well, maybe 'explode' is too strong a word. Banker Josh wasn't as exciting as that and I suspected he wouldn't be capable of making a social situation as dramatic as a bomb going off. The phrase 'a ticking time bomb yet to fizz' is probably more apt to describe the possibility of use bumping into each other in the future. The game was won that night but, cue the cheese, Josh hadn't won my heart. Next!

Guitarist_27

27 years old

6'3'' tall, average build

Northampton

Describe yourself…

I'm Bradley and I'm a photographer based in Northampton. I'm tall, friendly, with big blue eyes. I've just bought my own house - don't I feel grown up now lol!! I play lead guitar in a band – they're a good bunch, we've just started recording our first demo album. Wish us luck!

What are you looking for?

Good question. I don't think I'll know what I'm looking for until I find it!

A Chivalrous Man

Bradley and I decided to meet in a pub not far from my house, on the edge of a pretty conservation area, sliced in half by a river. Like many sunshine and Pimm's worshipers, pub gardens are definitely one of my favourite places to visit in the summer.

Bradley and I hit it off straight away. He was a lovely guy, with enthusiastic conversation on interesting and different topics to what I was used to. He talked photography, about his band (I will *not* become his groupie!), and a lot about his friends. It was a charming afternoon, no doubt helped by the turn of good weather. Even better news, there was definitely a bit of a spark between us. Hooray! I knew it was possible! I hoped this worked out slightly better than the initial spark I felt with Fabien…

Bradley let me choose where to base our second date, so I chose an old favourite of visiting the local 'pick your own'. We talked and laughed our way through picking over four large tubs of blackberries until our collection tubs were full, and, after a quick drink in the pub, he walked me home. I was feeling fantastic by this point. He was chivalrous, opening doors, showing interest by asking lots of questions about me, and he even made a point of walking street side of the pavement like a true gent. I liked that. He's obviously been brought up well.

Later that same week, Bradley invited me over to his place for dinner. I normally like to know what's for dinner, perhaps because of my mild phobia of finding an evil bean sprout on my plate or tasty some hideous cottage cheese. Happily, the beef casserole he produced was delicious and there was no sign of the aforementioned edible turn-offs. I brought the promised pudding round - a blackberry crumble I'd made with the berries we'd picked that past weekend. He loved it. He was totally smitten, it seemed, so I've included the winning recipe below – good luck baking!

Perhaps he was too smitten. Bradley was all in favour of quiet nights in, and had been mentioning about me meeting his band mates ('extended family') since our first date in the pub. This was all too cosy for me. I think the first few dates should be fun and involve lots of getting out-and-about together. There's plenty of time in the months to come for nights in with a DVD and hanging out with mutual friends. Plus, if someone keeps going on about how he *knows* I'd like his mates, it puts me off. Am I worried about being so predictable? No, I think I just don't like being told what I like. He certainly knew what he liked – being in a band, and me!

Anyway, the following Saturday night we rented a DVD and got a Chinese takeaway. It pretty much cemented my feelings on not wanting to spend our 'honeymoon' period cuddling on the couch. Don't get me wrong; although he was lovely and would truly have charmed the pants off my family, part of the puzzle was missing. I just felt he was too attached this early on, a bit soft, and I was a bit overwhelmed by it all. Let's have some fun getting to know each other before we start on meeting family, friends, and then progress upstairs from cuddling on the couch.

The next morning I decided I'd call him to end our relationship. There was something lacking with my and Bradley's, albeit short, relationship. Something came up though (honestly) and it slipped my mind. Sunday was a busy day for him anyway with band rehearsals and such like, so I decided it would be better to leave until the next day.

I came into work on the Monday wondering how to word the "you're dumped" conversation. It was long overdue now.

As I entered my office that morning, I saw a big box on my desk, delivered in the mail. A feeling of dread swept over me when I saw the return address - Bradley's house. How did he figure out my work's address? What had he sent me? And on the day I was planning on dumping him? Argh!

Inside the box was a real collection of treasures:

- ♥ three Crunchie chocolate bars (my favourite)
- ♥ four oranges - I'd been eating them like crazy on a health kick that week
- ♥ strawberry shoelaces - the only liquorice I will eat
- ♥ a chocolate orange (yum!)
- ♥ the Fortune Cookie I'd not eaten from the Chinese on Saturday night

How bad was I feeling right now? The poor guy had made such an effort, and if it had been someone I was honestly into, I would have truly been swept off my feet. Who doesn't enjoy personal packages delivered to your desk at work, let alone when it's full of your favourite snacks?

Feeling sick, I manned up and called Bradley at lunchtime to thank him for the box. Then came the killer punch – I explained it was all a little too much, and I wasn't sure our relationship had any ground we could run on. He was very nice about it all, which made it feel even worse, but I thought it was better to be honest, and I had put off dumping him for two days already.

Guilt! How bad did I feel?! I gave away a lot of the gifts in the box to people at work, which helped with the guilt a little. I threw the Fortune Cookie into the bin - I did NOT want to know what wise words that little snack had for me right now.

Louise's Adoration Inducing Fruit Crumble Recipe

(use with caution!)

Ingredients:

- 500g / 1 lb blackberries and apples (enough to fill your Pyrex dish)

- 150g / 6oz Sugar

- 1 teaspoon Cinnamon

For the topping:

- 150g / 6oz plain Flour

- 75g / 3oz Butter or Margarine

- 50 - 75g / 2 - 3oz Sugar

Time: 1 hour
Serves: 4

Instructions:

- Peel, core and slice the apples into slices and put into a 1 litre or 2 pint heatproof dish (Pyrex is good). Mix in the blackberries with the sugar.

- Mix flour in a bowl then rub in butter finely.

- Add sugar then toss lightly so the ingredients mix together.

- Sprinkle crumble over fruit thickly and evenly then press down softly with your palm

- Preheat the oven to 190 degrees centigrade, then bake for 15 minutes

- Reduce temperature down to 180 degrees centigrade and bake for a further 45 minutes, or until the top is a nice light golden brown colour.

- Remove and leave to cool before serving.

Serving Instructions:

- Serve with custard, double cream, fresh cream, or ice cream.

- Serve hot or cold

Joe5000

25 years old

5'7" tall, average build

Toronto, Canada

Describe yourself…

Welcome to my profile!

As you can see, I'm 25, a non-smoker, and I work for a finance firm in Toronto. A lot of my friends relocated back to the cities they studied in, so I'm left in the city in the market to meet some new people. I enjoy watching sports, especially baseball, love eating out, and I'm learning sign language at evening classes. If you want to say hi, I promise to reply!

What are you looking for?

A warm hearted woman who likes good conversation and a laugh.

Toblerone Toronto Joe

This date may seem a little chronologically unsound as Joe was my first internet 'meet', (and the only guy I have ever waited longer than 25 minutes for), but Joe fits perfectly into my 'having his own interests' tick box.

I was living in Canada at the time, waiting for my university friends to come back to town for the new school year. As the theme of the majority of my dating experience follows, Joe and I met on an international dating website. He made me a laugh during our lengthy, and conversation flowed beautifully. He seemed a nice enough guy so I decided to use his limited expertise in computers as an excuse for a casual meeting. He was far more clued up on computers than me, and I could use all the help I could get in fixing up my wireless internet.

We decided to go shopping for a wireless router for my new flat. That's why we met in the Futurshop PC store in St Catharines. Although I was soaked through from waiting in a rainstorm, I felt relaxed, maybe a tiny bit nervy. Toronto Joe was my first online date, but I wasn't too worried because the electronics superstore was a safe environment. I reassured myself I was playing 'at home' as we were meeting in my town and he didn't know the area – it makes it sound like I was planning a quick getaway, but you have to consider these things.

However, I knew I was just going to be myself and see where it led. There's no point being pessimistic about it, best to go in expecting success if I was going to take online dating seriously. I figured if Joe didn't show up I'd just depend on the sales people to help me buy the right router. Who knows, I might even pick up another hot electronics salesperson!

Joe was a little late, not knowing his way around the local area, but when he did arrive, Joe and I luckily got on like a house on fire. There was no need to put a quick exit plan into action. He was friendly, chilled out, and totally not fazed by the fact I'd known him less than three weeks and only by the e-waves. Maybe he was an old hand at this game…

We shopped, then I did something I thought I'd never do - I let him come back to the house I was temporarily living in and we… baked cakes! I'm normally pretty protective about my phone number and where I live for obvious reasons, but hey, I was moving house again in a week, he'd never know where to if it all went pear shaped. It was my friend's birthday the next day and the ridiculous American cooking conversions from grams into cups made for an interesting batch of cakes – first a concrete block, then a soggy mess, and finally, we nailed it with a perfect Toblerone flavoured cake.

Unfortunately for Joe, he wasn't my type, but we bonded over sugar highs and cakes built like bricks. We remain friends to this day. Joe says he'd chew his right arm off to date me, but now he's saved himself the pain of amputation by finding someone more suited to him.

BritishOli

23 years old

5'9" tall, athletic build

Hamilton, Canada

Describe yourself...

I'm half English, but I've lived in Canada since I was two years old. I enjoy in-line skating, and going out on the lake with my boat. My favourite food is Mexican, and sometime in the future I'd like to travel back to England to see the country my dad's family came from. I like rock music, barbeques, and hanging out with my friends. I don't like smokers, rap music or lentils.

What are you looking for?

A 20-something girl, who doesn't expect an English accent!

A British Pretender

Oli, Oli, Oli. This was another early internet date. We met in the car park of a local Canadian coffee house chain, Tim Horton's.

Sketchy? I should have guessed. We met under the pretence that it would be good to know another Brit in Canada, even though he was only half British...

We enjoyed a nice cup of coffee and planned to meet again. He seemed nice enough, so after work one night, we went in-line skating down the canal. We didn't stop for miles, and after exhausting ourselves, we crashed out on a grass bank and watched the stars – how romantic! He was a boat obsessed (own interests – check!) and a chemical engineer, so conversation was … slow… at points, as I know nothing about boats or chemicals, but by midnight I was exhausted, and went home having had a nice evening.

The next time I saw him was when he invited me to a pool party he was having that evening. Oli still lived with his mum, who had a pool in her garden, and I naively thought "*what fun*".

When we arrived at the front door, I noticed the big sailing boat in the driveway. The largest one they could squeeze onto their gravel driveway. Wow. This family sure liked boats.

Entering the house, clutching a bottle of wine I'd grabbed on the way over, it was unsettlingly quiet, no music or voices to be heard. There were hardly any lights on even. It was getting lat and it quickly became apparent that no one was invited to the party except me. I was pretty mad at myself for falling for that old trick! I had an immediate uncomfortable feeling, but Oli had not put a foot wrong yet so I decided to stick about for an hour or so and make my excuses.

We swam in the pool, it got a little bit romantic, and then it got weird. I had had enough by then. It was pretty late by then, but I had no idea where I was. I had no idea how to get out of his town and back to mine though because I'd followed him several miles out of town in my car and was new to the area. Plan B was the policy of just being polite and getting through the evening. After all, we'd had a good evening skating before, so there was every reason this might still work out. Still, lesson learnt – take a sat nav on any date out of town.

Oli offered his bed to me while he promised to sleep on the couch, but I spent the whole night fending him off. I should have jumped in the car and worked out the trip home in the dark myself. I didn't see Oli again.

Gut feelings – something to be said about that.

Written in the Stars

Just after I got back from holiday in Portugal last summer, I went wandering around town looking for furniture for the new place I was moving to in a couple of weeks. I still had lots of time, in no particular hurry, but thought I'd get an idea as to how much it might cost me to kit out my new, bigger bedroom. I'd passed by an independent sofa store hundreds of times before on my way into town, but this time I went on in intending to browse the bedroom cabinets.

I did browse, but, of course, I was looking for more than just household furnishings. You never know where you might strike lucky! I got chatting to the shop owner, Rhys. He was pretty cute at "about 35 years old" (so probably a little older…). We talked about my holiday, his holiday, my plans to move, and his daughter – ooh, a family man! I liked that instantly. I'd prefer to stay out of the 'children scene' until my 30's, but I could see there were some good sides to the prospect of me, a single woman with no kids, dating a dad.

√   He's a family man – a good quality in any bloke, one of my 'must-haves'. Maybe he'd be open to extending his family in the future…?

X   It's someone else's child – I'd probably have to share the responsibility on someone else's terms if Rhys and I got serious. What if our morals, upbringing methods and ideas of discipline were poles apart?

√   Something new to talk about, a learning opportunity – hah, I can foresee won't last long as a positive point!

X   He'd have a limited social calendar, reliant on babysitters and fitting enough 'Lou-time' around his daughter's dentist appointments, PTA meetings, ballet classes…

√ However, he is only a part-time dad. Rhys and the mother (sorry, almost wrote 'monster'!) of the child are still on speaking terms and share custody.

√ There's always sweets in the glove box of any decent dad's car!

I left Rhys's furniture shop finally, not having bought anything. Rhys still asked me for my phone number, with an offer of taking me out to dinner.

That was, unfortunately, the extent of the excitement. He was embarrassingly unapologetic about being 20 minutes late for our drinks date, with no explanation for his tardiness. He had my phone number, why hadn't he called? By the time Rhys arrived, I was sitting on my hands and swinging my legs on the bar stool like an idiot, approaching a state of tipsy-ness. I was already two drinks ahead of him. Ever noticed how much faster you drink when and if you're on your own?

After another drink, (that was four for me now), Rhys insisted on taking me across town for dinner. I wasn't sure about leaving my neighbourhood trapped in this stranger's car, but I knew the restaurant he wanted to eat at, and it had a lovely menu and a relaxed atmosphere. The toddler seat in the back of his Toyota also put me at ease a little. He couldn't be all *that* bad an evening companion. After all, someone somewhere had certainly entertained him far enough one night at least to conceive a child!

Unfortunately, Rhys' choice topic of conversation appeared to be fairly limited. He was seriously into astrology and star signs. Any bloke who believes that crap is not my kind of man, but then I suppose I should be grateful the subject wasn't pig breeding again. The overall evening wasn't too bad apart from the infuriating and embarrassing 20 minute wait at the start, but he wasn't my cup of tea really.

What did my grandmother always tell me? Don't talk to strangers. Anyway, Rhys took the problem of declining any more advances off my shoulders - he never texted me again. Meeting someone new probably wasn't mapped out in his horoscope that month.

M1_Commuter

26 years old

5'7" tall, average build

Milton Keynes

Describe yourself…

I qualified as a science teacher a year ago, and I'm enjoying it so far. It's a lot of work, but what other job gives you such a great summer break?? The kids are great and I love it when I see the penny drop over an idea I've explained to them. I'm from a large family and one day I'd like one of my own.

I enjoy going out to pubs and nightclubs, mostly ones that play chart and dance music. I do have a karaoke song of choice, but I don't know if it would be the right time to reveal that right now lol!

I make a mean roast dinner, I live with two mates in Milton Keynes, and I can …count to 20 in Mandarin. I'm running out of things to say – if you like what you've seen so far, send me an email! Happy searching…

What are you looking for?

Both my housemates are in long(ish) term relationships and I'd like to have someone to make me feel as happy as they seem.

Cute Butt Brett

Here's one example of someone underestimating their build. I wouldn't have classed Brett as an 'average', as he did on his profile. He was more 'extremely athletic'. Bingo! So, online profiles can be deceiving in a positive sense as well as setting you up for disappointment. Remember the aged photo I'd based my interest on with Banker Josh and the ice hockey date? It was definitely a nice surprise to see his bulging biceps and fantastic butt standing at the bar when I walked into TGI Friday's for our first date. He was, from then on, referred to as 'CBB' by me and my gossip girls... or Cute Butt Brett.

Our first date (yep, there were more to follow this time) was right after I got back from holiday - again. Are you spotting a theme? Brett and I enjoyed a dinner of spicy chicken wings and things were progressing very well. Brett paid me lots of attention all night and confirmed he was interested in taking things further with a textbook goodnight kiss when we parted company. Chicken wings with the company of a tasty man - a very delicious date. Top marks! I couldn't wait for the next date with Brett. Second dates don't happen that often, I'm starting to understand, so I was glad to be excited about this one.

Our second date was another meal out, this time at a nice Indian restaurant in town. I'd wanted to go there for a few months as it had a good reputation, and they didn't let us down. The meal was delicious and we had a great evening out. Things were going up and up with Brett. Apart from his obvious good look and athleticisms, he'd travelled widely and wanted to visit some of the same places as me in the future, Brett could hold a decent conversation, and he obviously loved his family and spoke quite a bit about his niece. I could tell Brett loved her to bits. He was shaping up to be a great example of the kind of man I wanted.

Date three: Brett helped me move house. Random? Yes, but I had to move, and that Saturday was the only day that week we could meet up due to a busy work schedule.

I still think date number three is borderline territory for showing random online dates where you live, but, as you can probably guess, I was feeling good about this guy. Plus, the new house wouldn't need the obligatory whizz-round tidy up to make sure no cobwebs were dangling over doorways, and nothing threatening would be poking out from underneath the fridge.

Bless his heart, Brett made my weekend by helping me 15 miles down the road that weekend, involving two solo trips in his

BMW – much bigger and more practical for moving house than my little Yaris. The new place was about 15 miles further away from Brett, but it was a perfect place, and a great excuse to get out of the Northampton United Nations bedsit. We both had cars, and 15 miles is not much more than a 10 minute trip, so it wasn't an issue. What a star Brett was! His muscles definitely helped too – I remember making a mental note to notch up my gym efforts to keep up with my six-pack owning (soon to be) boyfriend.

Christmas was fast approaching. We were spending it apart, as it was still early days in our relationship. All eventually went well gift-wise. The delivery of the radio controlled helicopter I'd bought him went a little wrong when it arrived in pieces, but I scored a manic replacement in time for December 25th. Brett bought me a beautiful silver necklace from Karen Millen. I felt like a princess. Ooh, Karen Millen - he'd outdone himself there. I'd never even glanced in that shop, let alone owned anything from it!

The day I returned from my family's festivities, Brett and I were invited to dinner at his parents' house on New Years Day for lunch.

"Meeting the family on New Year's Day, are you crazy???" I hear you exclaim. I'll have you know, I behaved myself very well the night before to prepare for it. Cocktail. Pint of water. Repeat. Success!

Brett's family were lovely people, very friendly and they cooked us a great curry. Brett, his little niece and I happily played with his parents' spaniels most of the afternoon. Things were feeling good and I was really made to feel welcome by the whole family.

I spoke to soon. Not even three weeks into the new year, everything changed. I went on a short break to Canada for a friend's wedding in and I came back to a grand dumping ceremony. Crystal balls are hard to come by, but maybe I should have seen this one sneaking up on me. Lately, there had been several cancelled dates and plans together had been changed at the last minute a couple of times this month. "Babysitting my niece" was the favourite excuse. Brett decided he couldn't last a weekend without any action with me when I was across 'The Pond' apparently. Oh well, he obviously wasn't good enough for me, as I wasn't good enough for him. The world 'sorry' rarely features in dumping rituals, but I wasn't sorry to see him leave.

Five days later, after a few days of the obligatory post-dumping 'moping around the house' ritual (much to my housemate Tom's disgust and annoyance), it was my birthday. Brett surfaced from his swamp and called me the day before to say he had some presents for me. He wondered if he could bring them over. I tried to convince him it wasn't a good idea as I clearly didn't want to see him again, but he was very insistent. Persistent. So, the next day he popped over with three parcels wrapped very prettily. One was a book on Egypt (where I'd visited and fallen in love with the week we'd met), another was a nice bottle of perfume, and the third present was a CD I'd wanted.

Was he feeling guilty? Did he just not want to waste a good present? Well, I won't ever know. I don't make a habit of staying in touch with men who end things between us. As rare as that is – I'm normally the 'dumper', not the 'dumpee'!

I gave my sister the CD, buried the expensive looking book deep in my book case, and put the perfume for sale on eBay. I made a pretty little £40 from its sale. I didn't want anything more to do with Brett. Every man has an inner jerk – it just takes longer for some to show the percentage of jerk quality they possess. I'm not one for man-rants, but I'm guessing most men are about 75% jerk. Brett was closer to the 100% mark than I'd expected, even if he was a family man in a muscly suit.

CountryMusicFanUK

24 years old

5'9" tall, average build

Dunstable

Describe yourself…

Tall dark and handsome! Haha just kidding – well, I'm definitely tall and dark, I'll leave you to decide if I'm handsome enough!

What are you looking for?

A woman to make my life complete – if she has the same interests that's great, but I quite often think opposites attract. If you're intrigued, you know where to find me!

A Family Affair

This one is one of my favourite dates, yet on the face of it, our first date story seems kind of weird. I have a certain soft spot for Irish men, and that fact probably went a long way into convincing me to go out with Ambrose. It was probably the promise of that sexy accent!

Apart from that, we both had the same questionable taste in music – country , so things started well. As most people who enjoy country music seem to be in their retirement years and/or living in North America, Ambrose and I were good company for each other. Right from the start he was giving off all the right signals, and he was always asking me lots of questions when he replied to my emails. That's always a good sign in my book. I thought we would be a good match if we ever got together for a date.

So, inevitably, we decided our first date would have to be to go and see a country music gig. It was a good idea, something fun and different, and, like the ice hockey game with Josh, it provided us with something to entertain us so conversation wasn't likely to dry up. The gig was in a Student Union bar in London. This normally would have been a little far for me to travel to from the Midlands for a first date, plus Taylor Swift wasn't one of my favourite singers, but hey, American country music doesn't come to the UK very often so it had to be worth supporting. Plus there was the lure of Ambrose's accent to tempt me!

Gig dates – pros and cons...

√   Something in common to talk about. Although, the loud music isn't exactly conducive to free-flowing conversation. How many times can you say "pardon?" and "sorry?" without bawling at each other? Nodding and smiling to whatever your date says follows...

√   You get to listen to some live music. I'm assuming you both had some say in which gig you'd attend together so one of you wasn't in agony all evening listening to an unknown rap collective when you were expecting Lady Gaga

X   Being surrounded by crowds, there's no chance at all of any first date intimacy

√   You could be pressed up close to your date all evening. Hot! But, wait, this could easily be a distinct disadvantage too – you'd better hope he wore deodorant that evening!

X   Going to a gig's not a cheap date once you've bought concert tickets/train tickets/drinks etc – make sure you choose a gig you'll enjoy!

√   You can drink, dance and let your hair down. But keep a lid on it, you don't want to scare him off

The weird thing about this particular date was that Ambrose's mum and sister were coming with us. As big Taylor Swift fans, they'd too bought tickets. Awkward! However, I decided to take it as a good thing that they were present because it meant that:

a) Ambrose wasn't shy about his family meeting me
b) He probably had already told them he'd met me online
c) I tend to like men who get along their families – unlike Ashley in the "Films and Music" chapter soon to follow!

Plus, having the family there kind of took the pressure off it being a date scenario and we could just enjoy the gig. It would give us something to talk about if a second date materialised too. What a story for the potential kids should things work out – "Your nan came on our first date!" Imagine their faces, how archaic to have a chaperone!

Despite my slight reservations, the gig was a lot of fun, and the music was better than expected. Taylor Swift seemed lovely and looked like she was genuinely enjoyed playing her debut UK gig. After having a such a wonderful night out, I didn't expect the evening to finish so abruptly. Ambrose (and his family) and I accidentally got on opposite escalators at the Tube Station without realising to make our respective journeys home on the trains. As the moving staircases transported us further apart, we shared an awkward smile and wave. Very strange.

'Goodbye, then!' I thought. Ah, he'd call if he wanted to see me again. I wasn't going to chase after him that's for sure.

Fast forward a year or so, and Ambrose is seeing someone else now. Since our date, we've slowly evolved into being good friends, and at the time of writing, Ambrose and I are an hour away from going shopping together for fancy dress costumes for Halloween.

Ambrose was definitely one of my most memorable first dates, even though it was never anything romantic. Perhaps I should have guessed it wasn't going to blossom into the romance of the century. I mean, who brings their mum along on a first date? I would have been embarrassed to suggest the idea to anyone I'd hooked for a date. Well, I guess, in fairness, Ambrose didn't warn me beforehand. I learnt my lesson fast here (in fact, the minute I walked into the venue and saw the family with Ambrose), but our 'date' wasn't a complete disaster at least.

Spy Mission!

Tempted to begin her own quest to find a man, Jenn, a friend of mine, and I decided one day to go on a 'spy mission' on a local singles night. We thought it was a good idea to find the details of a local 'meet' from one of the sites we were registered on, and go undercover to suss out the talent/competition.

This particular evening was planned as a bowling event for people from Milton Keynes, aged between 20 and 40 years old. Jenn and I figured as a pair there was safety in numbers and we headed down to the bowling alley complex just before the dates were due to arrive. We settled on a couple of comfy bar stools with a full view of the bowling lanes and bar area.

Enter the contestants! There seemed to be a wide-ish range of people attending in terms of age and appearance, and there were some potentials we felt we might have wanted to approach for a chat, if we were there on official dating 'business'. They looked like they were having a good time, relaxing, drinking, and bowling, and it gave us a much needed confidence boost in the online dating scene, as well as a great giggle for single ladies like us, watching the scene unravel.

There were about 16 people in attendance, but there was a ratio of about three women for every man. That was far from ideal, but we came away thinking we might have the guts to go to another event properly now we've scoped it out (see the chapter on 'rugged good looks'). With hindsight, we probably should have swooped in on those unsuspecting singles and chatted them up posing as innocent bystanders, allegedly unaware that it was a singles' night out. Maybe next time. That takes some serious guts!

Now where am I on the check list? Ah, the chapter regarding my search for a man with intelligence. Let's see how this works out…

The Grass Isn't Always Greener

One evening, in the spring of the year I lived in Northampton, my friend Rachel and I went out for a night on the tiles, sampling all the dilapidated delights of the town. On our way home, I thought I heard someone calling my name behind me, through the crowd of drunken and stumbling party goers. '*Very strange*' I thought, as I hadn't been living in Northampton long, and no one really knew me. They must be after someone else.

The calling got more earnest and I turned on my heel. Ok, not so slick – I turned on the heel of my sparkly shoes with a little stumble, a result of several fruity cocktails. There stood a man with a shaved head, most definitely beckoning to me.

"It *is* you!" he said, grinning from ear to ear. "I'm Phil." Phil extended his arm and shook my hand.

Phil. Phil, Phil, Phil. I racked my brains thinking, '*how do I know this guy?*' Well, the only thing was to ask. I still wasn't convinced he'd got the right Louise.

"Umm… sorry… Phil. Do I know you?"

He laughed, a friendly deep laugh. "Well, no, not really. I've seen you on Facebook and thought I recognised you just now." Had he been trawling the internet looking for younger women? Creepy! It's more than a little weird when a bloke peruses online potential from a non-dating website like Facebook. I'd have to check my privacy settings again.

"You're on the same environmental network page as me." Rings a bell... How did he remember me from possibly hundreds on such a website?

"Riiiiight…" I said, giving my friend a get-me-out-of-here look. "Great! Have a good night!"

And with that, Rachel and I jumped into a cab and headed home.

*   *   *

Two days later, I received a message from Phil through Facebook, inviting me to the next meeting of Northampton's

Greenpeace group, since he knew I had keen, green environmental interests at my very core. Greenpeace would not be my first choice of environmental group to join, which should have been my first reason not to go, but I went along anyway. I was looking for something to do that night, I was looking to meet more people in my new location, and it could be interesting. You never know!

Well, it wasn't – well, not interesting in terms of the Agenda to be discussed, but the mixed bag of people in attendance provided all the free entertainment I needed for that evening. We set the environmental world to rights from 7pm, sitting in a dingy, slightly whiffy pub in Abington. The leather stool seats had rips in the upholstery, and the windows needed a good clean. Although the drink was cheap, I wouldn't have gone back there for any social occasion.

The small group of environmentalists vaguely discussed environmental matters and ways forward to influence the great and the (not so) good. I was welcomed by a young hippy who looked liked she'd made her skirt from a selection of men's ties. There was also a seemingly mad man in his late 70's who kept asking if the pub was closing, and old and odd couple who were proud to be the longest standing members and who seemed to be the most intelligent and the most active politically. And, of course, there was Phil.

I was looking forward to the end of the meeting after a couple of minutes of it having started, thinking this group was stuck in it's old ways and hadn't learnt anything new about the environment and protecting it since the mid-1980's. I was also increasingly worried I might turn into one of these oddballs should I linger any longer.

When they asked me my opinion on the construction of wind turbine farms, my positive and not uncommon opinion was met with a stony silence. A true tumbleweed moment. Save me.

When conversation began again (on a different subject), I caught Phil muffling a laugh. His eyes were shining and giggling behind his pint. I rolled my eyes at him, sharing the joke of the ancient and dope smoking fuddy-duddies we shared company with, and got myself another drink.

Two hours later, and the meeting had long been adjourned. Phil and I were having a good laugh about the evening's humble events and the characters present. Nothing spiteful, I think he was just tired of the same old faces and political inaction, and was grateful for a fresh face and new perspective. He seemed proactive and keen on helping preserve the environment, and he knew more about protecting it for the future than all of my colleagues and friends combined. We had a lot to talk about.

Phil came across as intelligent, working as a radiotherapist, and was full of smiles. I like than in a man. You can tell if a smile's genuine and this one was. He was Bletchley born and bred, single, (yes, I'd assumed that!), although he had been married and divorced when he was younger. Well, he actually said "young", but no warning bells rung at this point for me. I need to get them fine tuned at some point… We had had a bit of a laugh that evening in Abington, but he was a little older than guys I'd dated before… 35? 37 years old maybe?

When I returned home, there was already a message waiting for me in my Facebook inbox. He liked his social media, that was certain! I hoped he had a mobile phone… The message contained another invitation to dinner. Could I join Phil for dinner tomorrow night? I did consider this carefully. He was a vegetarian, and in my view that's not an attractive attribute in a potential couple where one of them, me, likes to cook. I do *not* want to get into the situation where I'm having to rustle up two separate meals every evening, one veggie, one carnivorous. Anyway, that was potentially a long way into the future, so I took Phil up on his offer. Well, what did I have to lose? I let him wine and dine me in a lovely little place hidden away in a village between Northampton and Milton Keynes. We enjoyed a relaxing meal, nothing overly romantic, and it was really rather nice. I realised I'd gotten used to being treated a little less special (case in point, TV Jake), and was enjoying the relative 'poshness' of the restaurant. I might have to make a point of demanding a little more from future dates. I deserve better than Wetherspoons (Fabien!). Maybe the older man was the way forward… We had a little smooch at the end of the night, and I wasn't disappointed, but had to wipe a little juice off my face. Spray guard anyone? We could work on that!

That evening, Phil and I were increasingly flirty on text. I was careful enough, aloof but accessible – texts are as un-doable as a tattoo, I have learnt. I had followed this mantra and hadn't sent any drunken messages for, ooh, about three weeks now. I won't bore you with the detail of our conversation, but he did pipe up towards the end of our conversation with one gem: "How old do you think I am?"

Now, I am notoriously crap at guessing people's ages, but I think I thought I had my finger on the pulse with this one. I knew he was older, but there couldn't be *that* much of an age difference between us. We'd had such a nice evening out together after all.

I replied playfully, "how old do you think *I* am?"

He was almost bang on, only two years older my 23 years. Good guess. I, however, was way off. He wasn't in his mid-to-late 30's. He was almost double my age, at 44 years old. Secretly, my initial reaction was "EWW!!!" but then I remembered how much fun we'd had together so far. We wound up our conversation, and I went to bed that night feeling a little cautious, but a little excited too. Here was a type of man I'd never met before, something new, and hopefully something good. I wasn't sure how long his attentions (or mine!) would last, but I thought I'd see how it went. Does age really matter after all? If only he could kiss with a little less spray. I'd like to keep my makeup intact if possible!

A couple of proper dates followed - no more Greenpeace meetings, thank God! We had dinner at a true Italian pizza parlour in Bletchley, and enjoyed a lively rugby match at The Saint's ground in Northampton. One of the more inventive dates we had was the 'Yellow Pages Date'.

What's that? You've never heard of a 'Yellow Pages Date'?! Well, I don't blame you for not knowing what one of these are, as I think I may have the claim on inventing it! It's a winning formula for when your inspiration for new date locations are running low. Fear not, it's no secret, here's your step-by-step guide.

The Yellow Pages Date Formula

Step 1. Find a copy of your local Yellow Pages. You have it somewhere…

Step 2. One of you (the couple) flicks through the pub section like you would a cartoon animation flick book and the other person hollers "STOP!" at some random point.

Step 3. The first person then closes their eyes and points with their finger to somewhere on the open page.

That's the pub you will head to for drinks tonight – have fun!

Our 'Yellow Pages Date' was a particularly successful one We ended up in a working men's club on the south side of town, where the drinks were oh so cheap as chips. Always a winner! Inside, I was preparing myself to manning up to break the news I was dating such an older guy to my family and friends. One more date needs to cement the deal before I drop that particular middle-aged bomb, I think…

The best date we had in that short three week period of testing out our compatibility was when we went for a long walk over the hills and fields near Bedford, hiking and hunting down wind turbines. I'd never seen one live in the flesh, (well, in shiny white metal), so I loved it. Reminiscent of the first Greenpeace meeting where Phil and I made our first connection, they were enormous but so much quieter than I'd imagined. Hah, I knew being pro-turbine was the right decision!

We wove our way into a village for a pub lunch, and we sang our hearts out on the journey home along to the new The Killers CD he'd brought along for the ride in his shiny Toyota Prius. How environmentally friendly! I was amazed at the common ground between us and how well I held my own in the environmental debates and discussions we had on the way home.

When we got back to his place to retrieve my car, we went inside for a cup of tea. That's when things started to get a bit serious. Phil and I made our way upstairs and things progressed into the bedroom. I don't remember exactly what happened next, but I think I mentioned I wanted to take things slowly.

Note my sarcasm here - what an insult. Phil didn't like that one bit. A mixture of a growl and a yell shot right into my face, and he threw me down onto the mattress. I started to struggle, trying to wiggle away from him. He grabbed me by the throat and hollered "What can I do to please you?! You've been winding me up all day!"

I made him recoil by doing something I'd never do to someone I truly loved and felt comfortable with. I kicked him in the balls. I would find it hard to do to a stranger! I was totally confused - where had this angry explosion come from? We'd had a lovely day out, I thought. Shocked and more than a little scared, I leapt off the bed, grabbed my things and jumped into my car. Hands shaking, I started the engine and quickly drove off. I didn't reach the end of his road before I was crying from shock and relief, but I kept driving.

*   *   *

The following evening, feeling a little sorry for myself, I was wrapped up warm and safe in my duvet. I'd been glad not to hear from Phil since that horrible evening at his house. It was a DVD night in, and I was enjoying lazing about in my bedroom with my relatively 'new' charity shop TV.

It was around 8pm when the doorbell went. One of my housemates answered it. It was Phil. He had come over with not one, but two bunches of flowers, and I know he hates cut flowers - so un-environmentally friendly. He'd told me before he'd only normally buy a potted plant, for longevity. He must be trying to make an effort. Hah, you can try, good luck to you!

I asked him why he was here, because I didn't want to see him. He replied he wanted to say sorry. Was he smirking a little? I wasn't sure. I looked around the living room where we were awkwardly standing. Had my housemate made herself scarce already?! Great.

Ok, so he's sorry. Not forgiven.

"I brought you flowers…" he pleaded with a hint of a whine.

"Why have you brought *two* bunches of flowers?" I enquired.

"In case I've done something else wrong I'm not aware of."

Jackass. What a prat. Phil didn't even know what he'd done wrong and thought two wilting bunches of petrol station forecourt flowers would make up for whatever he did, whether he was aware of how horrific his behaviour had been. Who knows, maybe he thought acting that much of a thug was normal dating practice?

I took the flowers from him, said thank you (as all polite girls should), and closed the front door, leaving him looking confused on the doorstep. *'Don't come back'* I thought.

Almost a year later Phil tried to contact me by text, a message spoken as if we were long-lost friends who needed to touch base again. I didn't recognise his number, having deleted all contact details from this man, but he revealed it was my "eco friend from Bletchley", and I did not reply. That was the last I heard from Phil. He might have ticked my 'intelligent' box but if I saw him again, it would be too soon.

Since then, (but not as a consequence of this encounter), I have become less 'green' minded. Phil can't credit himself with even that. Toyota Prius's are ugly, I don't want my man to have so many similar common interests as me as you end up talking about the same stuff all the time, and I'd rather go out with a guy with a more gentle lime green soul than dark green one.

A Keen Man at The Green Man

Manchurian Mark, despite his northern accent, was a guy from a small town in the Midlands, not too far from me. He'd moved there several years ago and I was surprised to find someone online who knew of my small village. An instant ice breaker. We went for a drink at The Green Man pub one evening. It was an odd place to go for a first date, with hindsight. I mean, it was ok - friendly, clean, cheap, easy to get to, but it was more of a truck stop pub for passing trade, as it's on a main trunk road snaking through Northamptonshire.

As I expected from our frequent chats online, we did get along well. Mark seemed intelligent, chatty, and we had a similar education. Mark was indeed a nice guy, although he was nothing like his profile picture in the flesh. I think I should ask to see more than one picture in the future before any date plans are made…

Ah, the wisdom of experience. The chances of the guys actually looking like their picture have got to be much more likely if you see more than one image. I like to chat with a webcam too (if only briefly, they're suspicious gadgets), as there is no question then if they're a sixty year old man with elasticised trousers and a cigar posing as a tall, dark and handsome twenty-something.

I wondered if Mark was quickly falling into the 'friend' category right from our first 15 minutes together, just like Joe from the computer shop date in Canada. So, when he asked me out on another drink I went along with it, since we had a pleasant enough evening at The Green Man. However, I remorsefully regretted this when Mark texted me later to say he was mad at himself for not kissing me.

'Why ruin an enjoyable evening by having to fend a girl off', was my immediate thought.

He may be smart but Mark hadn't sensed I'd not been that into him. I knew it was all feeling rather wrong and ended it there, feeling I was sailing too close to the wind in terms of leading him on. It's a bad sign if you can't picture yourself kissing your date back when they're pretty keen.

Unfortunately, I am reminded almost every day of that awkward conversation over why I didn't want to see him like that anymore, as Mark has what would pass for as an evil twin who goes to the same gym as me. Damn.

However, this goes to show that not all my encounters were awful, naughty-in-a-bad-way, or with criminally, morally or financially questionable people. Mark only encouraged me to carry on, and led me to increase my efforts of searching for the perfect date.

TRN27

27 years old

5'11'' tall, athletic build

Milton Keynes

Describe yourself…

I work for an accounting firm in Milton Keynes. I went to university in Sheffield and I like to spend my weekends making the most of my time off. I am friendly, chatty, honest, and I have an open mind about most things. My friend put me up online for a joke, but I think secretly that she'll be eating her words if I find "the one"! I am definitely a "dog" person – no "cat" people may apply!!! (Joke… kind of!!)

What are you looking for?

I'm open to suggestions…

My Funny Valentine

This is a pretty short story. The decision to meet up with Terry was a last minute one, as we'd only been talking, at best, for three days. The fourth day was Valentine's Day and neither of us had any romantic rendezvous planned that night. In a move fuelled by loneliness, boredom and curiosity, we thought what's the harm in meeting for a drink? No harm at all, we'd keep it uncomplicated and casual, a 'non-date'.

'Non-dates' – pros and cons...

√ No pressure, no rules – just friends going for a drink

√ You can do non-traditional date activities like shopping – much like Toronto Joe, and *that* date was an unexpected success in a meeting a new friend

√ If it all goes horribly wrong, no one loses face or loses out, and no one gets the wrong idea

X Time and energy invested into making sure it's definitely not a date seems wasted when you could be on a *real* date. What's the point???

Anyway, aide from all of that, Terry and I at least both ended up getting reasonable no-pressure company for the stupidly auspicious day of Valentine.

I can't fault the pub. The drinks weren't ramped up to Valentines Day prices and the atmosphere was warm and inviting. I particularly liked the comfy leather sofas. '*They'd go well in my living room*', I mused as I walked into the bar.

Terry, however, turned out not to be my type – a little on the camp side. In my defence and before you tell me off for being closed-minded and fussy, Terry actually got approached in the pub toilets that night by a man, so you get the idea. As you might expect, nothing really developed from our evening together. Good job it wasn't a real date then!

We did, until recently, still say hi occasionally if we bumped into each other in town. It seemed we were on the same bar circuit. However, things took a much colder turn though recently when Terry saw me, absolutely wasted, talking to another guy in a club one night. He went off in a strop and I never heard from him again.

The Return of the Repaired Laptop

With Housemate Tom lending me a replacement computer for the time being, and one thing and another keeping me busy (well, let's be more specific - Bradley, Brett, Ambrose, Terry...), I didn't collect my laptop from the repair shop for a couple of weeks. I eventually popped into the shop on a Friday after work and found Max manning the fort alone again.

"Sorry I've left it so long", I said.

"It's fine, we have a large storage cupboard", Max winked. "People are so busy nowadays". Little did he know just *how* busy I'd been…

The number one song in the UK charts suddenly sounded out in a tinny multi-tonal ringtone. Max grabbed his handset off the desk. "You don't mind do you?" he said, raising his eyebrows. "It's my brother and we're planning a surprise knee's up for my mum's 50th tonight."

I nodded, waving him on. Poor bloke, organising a family do. How complicated do you think it could be getting all your relatives happily in the same room for a couple of drinks? Very complicated, is the answer. I sympathised - I'd attempted something similar a couple of months before for my own family.

Busying myself by pretending to look at the PC accessories display to the right of the service counter, I didn't have to wait long. I smiled away Max's apologies for the interruption.

"It seems you've got it all in hand. I hope your mum enjoys herself tonight."

"Yeah, I hope it all turns out ok," he nodded. "I'm not sure how she'll react to the surprise but it'll be good to see everyone together for once." Any fool could tell he was looking forward to the evening. It was nice to see. So many people spend their lives escaping their family, and it's an endearing quality in a man. Wait, isn't that on my checklist? He must be a local too, working in a shop only 10 minutes from my house. Interesting…

Anyway, I paid for the computer repair, a smaller hit in the purse than what I'd expected. It seems the problem was an easy fix – a man with computer intelligence is invaluable! I'd recommend this shop anytime! One happy customer.

Later that evening I thought of Max and his family and their birthday 'knee's up'. I'd never know how it went, but I quietly hoped it was all Max had planned for. He seemed nice, and deserved to have a great weekend.

Dylan_Dimebar

25 years old

5'9'' tall, slim build

Milton Keynes

Describe yourself…

I enjoy hiking, reading, and cooking – you should try my lasagne! My favourite first date would be something where we could chat (the cinema is a bit useless for that!) and we can have some fun. Have you tried ice skating before? I'm a fun-loving guy who's honest and caring. What more could you ask for?

What are you looking for?

To be honest, this is a "last hurrah" for me on this website, I'm finding it all too much like hard work! I'm looking for that special person and don't want to be messed about. If you're interested, you know how to get in touch!

Dylan cropped up as a potential online date after I had a bit of a break from the whole online dating scene. Although glad to have my laptop back, I'd thought by this time that most online dates were in fact a waste of time and I'd had enough. However, Dylan seemed like a catch when he popped up as a 'recommended for you' candidate on the website. So he and I arranged to meet one Friday night at the tenpin bowling centre. We would have been talking online every day via email or instant messaging a few weeks by then, and bowling is always a good first date activity I think.

Bowling – pros and cons...

√   A chance to talk and to have a giggle

X   Like the concert date with Irish Ambrose, there was no chance at all of any first date intimacy – a party of screaming 10 year olds in the lane next to you is hardly a turn-on

√   You can work out if he's ultra competitive – be that a good or bad trait in your opinion – and seeing if he can take losing like a man

X   Or, on the flipside, you might show you're not able to take the embarrassment following the whipping he gave you with his impressive score of strikes

√   In a bowling alley, it's easy to avoid the alcohol if your tongue gets a bit loose after a couple of vinos.

So 7pm rolled round on that Friday night and I showed up on the dot. I was a little anxious as I approached the entrance to the bowling alley. Would I be too short, too tall? Too fat or too skinny? Too overdressed, underdressed, or would I just be too chatty for him? I had high hopes for this date and didn't want anything to go wrong.

I caught the eye of a tall, dark haired man loitering at the bowling alley's entrance. He made a half smile, confirming it was Dylan. As I approached, I thought quietly "Ermm... great - he looks a lot older in the flesh", but it was too late now.

"You must be Dylan" I said with a forced smile. "I'm Louise".

"Yes", he replied, "nice to meet you", and we began walking into the bowling centre.

Just as I was planning the first moves on my get-out excuse, maybe midway through our first game, I felt a tap on my shoulder. Dylan carried on walking in, and I turned round to see who wanted my attention. It was… Dylan! The real Dylan. The photo fit was perfect from his profile pictures (gorgeous!), and definitely younger that the impersonator who was leading me off.

Feeling a bit of a fool, I can't even remember what I mumbled to the original 'Dylan' and quickly walked inside with the real thing. I don't know what Dylan no.1 was thinking – maybe he was on an internet date himself and mistook me for his date, or possibly he even thought I was a better option. Maybe he'd organised a blind date, but that seemed quite a coincidence… This date of his, if indeed it existed, obviously had the same name as me. Or perhaps he'd not heard me correctly when I introduce myself? Why would he pretend to be called Dylan? Or maybe he *was* named Dylan, and I'd come across the most incredible coincidence known to man. Probably not, he was probably just a dirty old man. What a lucky escape!

Anyway, although I was morbidly horrified at my mistake, the real Dylan and I did manage to laugh about it all, and he was told-off light-heartedly by me for being late enough for another man to steal me away. Bowling, as expected, turned out to be lots of fun, and he didn't win by too big a margin. I was impressed with myself. God knows how the might have ended if I'd gone off with the fraudster.

Date two was fun as well. I enjoyed both Dylan's company and the food at my favourite South American themed restaurant Incidentally, it's not far from Albanian Arben's old place of work, I might add, but I wasn't going to linger in the forecourt chancing he or his cousin would see me. I'd so moved on! The most amusing moment of my date with Dylan was when dessert came – a messy dish of caramelised mini bananas in toffee sauce. They looked like a palm spread of fingers. Or something phallic… He was excellent company and obviously he enjoyed having a manly but frequent giggle. Very encouraging!

That night was particularly blustery and the wind tunnel effect in the car park really didn't help my carefully planned out outfit of a flowing skirt and hair recklessly unpinned on the walk back to our vehicles. We parted company with smiles on our faces though - a shy kiss from Dylan felt good, even if his longer-than-average goatee did tickle my nose into a expression strong enough to contend for the gold medal in a gurning competition.

Consequently date three was arranged shortly afterwards – hooray, he agreed to blackberry picking along the river. Fruit picking was a great first date idea I'd enjoyed previously with Bradley, so I tried it again. It worked like a charm. As I had the most disgusting symptoms of hay fever, I'm surprised Dylan wanted to even look at me, let alone arrange for a fourth date.

Date four involved Dylan cooking a lovely meal for me at his flat. Wow, date four, he's going the distance! With full bellies, we settled on his comfy sofa with a glass of wine each to watch *'The Last Samurai'* on DVD.

By the end of the film, however, I'd long lost any interest in Dylan, and Tom Cruise as well. What a pair of wet fish! I was convinced by the end of the evening Dylan didn't know what he was doing in the girlfriend department. I didn't want an inexperienced bloke I had to drag out of his shell. I'd had more excitement from my phone being set to vibrate. I rang him the following day to let him know I didn't think things were going to work out too well for us. I felt awful, he'd really not been a bad date at all, beautifully rugged, and we'd had fun. He just didn't have enough Pure Man Quality for me. Too harsh? Maybe.

*   *   *

Anyway, two weeks passed quietly, and a hand-delivered letter arrived on my doorstep. It was from Dylan. My heart dropped. Had he not got the message? Now, as a writer, I'm obviously not against people expressing themselves on paper, and some might think 'how romantic', but this move was a little akin to activities of a stalker. I didn't think I'd even told him where I lived...

Dylan spent his pages (plural!) proclaiming his love for me and reminiscing about the four 'fantastic' dates we'd had. A case of mistaken identity? A wind swept banana flavoured mess? A snotty, sneezy walk? Maybe *he* should be the one writing a book on bad dates if he thinks ours were so ground breaking.

That's mean. But, let's go back to the letter. It was a very amorous letter, especially considering I'd ended things between us a fortnight ago. If it had been from someone I wanted to be with I would have wooed to maximum levels, I am sure! Dylan ended the gushing four page letter with:

"If you have changed your mind and you'd like to see me again, I will be in Waterstones book shop at 4pm on Tuesday. I hope to see you there."

I imagined him standing in Waterstones on Tuesday, perhaps between the erotic fiction and the travel books, hiding behind a newspaper, wearing a bright carnation so I could spot him. However tempted I was to grab my passport and flee the country, there were a couple of problems with his Humphrey Bogart style plan. Firstly I worked until 5pm every day, so the timing was impossible for me, and secondly, and most importantly, I still hadn't changed my mind. Plus, what man of 25 years has granny-style flower scented writing paper? As handsome as Dylan was, things weren't going to work out. I sent him a quick text thanking him for the lovely letter, but no, I had not changed my mind, sorry.

Goldfield83

26 years old

5'10" tall, athletic build

Aylesbury

Describe yourself…

I like to treat my friends and family well, I like beach holidays, and I love my Mac Book! I'm an Ibiza-loving, sun worshipping clubber, who one day wants to live in the Mediterranean. I'm a vet, and I hope one day to open my own practice.

What are you looking for?

Someone who can keep up with my zest for life!

Vetting the Vet

Goldfield83 - he's a vet? Pull the other one! Everyone knows certain professions make women go weak at the knees, and a vet is one of them. Fortunately, I'm not one of the easily fooled, and I saw right through it. How did this vet afford the huge watch on his arm? The weight of his Rolex might explain the size of his biceps at least…

Anyway, Jeff turned out to be in alcoholic drinks marketing, and an awkward and despondent date who came back to bite me. From his hot but seemingly professionally posed photos on his profile, I knew he was a stylish man who spent time on his appearance. That's not normally my type, as I tend to prefer the more rugged, scruffy look, but what the hell, good looking is good looking - all types may apply, and indeed do. So, to try to give a matching faked stylish impression, I chose to wear a lovely summers dress to our pub garden date, purchased just for the occasion.

Our date didn't start well - I got lost on the way to the pub as I'd not visited Aylesbury before. When I showed up 20 minutes late, full of apologies, I found I was way too dressed up for the occasion. I felt a right numpty from the word go. Even in my favourite beaded flip flops and my stunning new dress. It wasn't a black tie cocktail dress or anything too fancy, but Jeff was in his "scruffs". Not a great sign – a man should make more of an effort! But, annoyingly, he looked great for his down-grade to holey jeans and a polo shirt.

To add to the problem, I was coming down with a cold and he was clearly hung over from whatever he got up to the night before. It didn't bode well for a successful date. It was a pretty painful affair, one I don't mean to repeat. It was clear neither of us really were in the right frame of mind, or even that interested in each other. He didn't seem to have much conversation in him, whether he was bored, too hung over, or disappointed in how I turned out in the flesh, I will never know, but I think he thought he was too good for me. Hunky, handsome, rugged 'vet' Jeff didn't call me again. No skin off my nose… Next!

*   *   *

Many more dates with other blokes and a whole year later, another guy and I had plans to go to the cinema. He was running late so I joined the ticket queue alone and intending to grab a pair of tickets before they sold out. Not far from the front of the line, I happened to glance around me and who was standing four people behind me? Jeff. Brilliant. I was not only trapped in the line, standing inches away from a guy who'd not deemed me worth another date, I was alone. Alone in the cinema queue. He was with a crowd of blokes. How sad, single and lonely must I have looked?

I kept my head down until I finally reached the ticket counter. The air con in the cinema did nothing to keep me cool, I was sweating buckets! How attractive. Anxiety peaking, I loudly announced I'd like TWO tickets for the next showing, hoping if Jeff had in fact clocked me he'd hear for sure that I was not going to the cinema on my own, still single.

Once the tickets were in my hand I quickly marched off to the toilets to text my late date a serious "hurry up!" message and waited. How silly, things like that don't normally make me nervous, but I did not want to run into Jeff and his friends again in the lobby.

My date eventually arrived (cutting it fine for the start of the film I may add!) and I left the safety of the ladies' toilets – just as Jeff was passing by on his way to the popcorn stand. No word of a lie. It was perfect timing, hey? I confessed to my date what happened, which he found hilarious. Looking back now, it was a pretty funny situation to be caught in. I wonder if Jeff did in fact see me queuing all on my own, or was it all in my paranoid imagination… Oh, and my late cinema date? He was alright, but the date was nothing momentous enough to document. Great film, average date who didn't materialise into anything exciting. Who's next?

Singles' Night - Part One

Wow, did this take some courage! My fellow online dating friend Jenn, from the previous bowling alley Spy Mission experience, and I registered for a singles' night 'group meet' which the dating website I belonged to had organised for members in Milton Keynes. We did it mainly for a laugh, but definitely out of quite a lot of curiosity and with quite a bit of hope too, especially since our successful snoop at the bowling alley a month or two back.

The bar all us singles were all supposed to meet in was located on the edge of the Milton Keynes Willen Lakes recreation park. It's a lovely lakeside setting, especially on a clear but cool night. I had never been to that bar before, and it was packed to the rafters. We were like single fish in a barrel. There had to be some potential in there somewhere!

As a bonus, it did appear to have a good ratio of men to women - spot on! Attendees from the dating site had to wear these hideous badges to identify other 'fish in the sea'. We both declined gracefully, perhaps mistakenly playing it a little too cool, and we claimed our territory on a comfy leather couch with a panoramic view of the bar. Every person in the bar looked dead nervous and most were coyly standing in single sex groups, just like in a school playground. We couldn't wait for the drinks to start melting the ice…

No one really that interesting approached us, although a weird looking guy in a duffel coat sat down next to me and then said nothing. He just stared into his pint glass. Maybe he'd not realised his local was hosting a singles' night and just wanted some peace. Poor chap!

Jenn and I decided we had had enough of window shopping, becoming more confident as the crowd seemed to be warming up, aided by the flowing liquor. It was an odd scenario, but knowing (assuming) the majority of the people in the buzzing bar were single, we began to mingle…

After closer observation, the bar was filled with slightly more women than men, I seem to remember, but like I said before, it had to be a pretty close ratio. It was better than I had expected, as I think more women attend these things than men in general. The men were on average a lot older than I'd have liked, but hell, I'll talk to anyone. I'm a conversation floozy. Cue a boring bus conductor, an overly confident (drunk?) man in his retirement years, and a biker clad in his full leathers. Maybe that was a subconscious protection ploy against all the single women… It occurred to me that perhaps it's better to hand pick people off a website than plunge into a singles' night because you can root out the ones who don't appeal straight away.

However, all was not lost. I did get talking to one guy, Karl, a gym instructor from Northampton. He was definitely the best looking bloke there in my opinion, and definitely the right side of 30. I could see his muscles through his well-chosen shirt, and there were the beginnings of some evening stubble appearing on his chin. Yum! After chatting a while, we swapped numbers and made a date a week later to go for a drink in a country pub. Success!

It was close to the end of the night so we reluctantly called it a day. I watched him leave the bar, my eyes lingering a little too long on the beautiful shape of his behind. I saw him get into a shiny black Audi. Now that's nice. I am not into flashy cars in general, but Pig Farmer Lewis has taught me to be a little more discerning on the matter. I have learnt to appreciate a nice model – oh, and a good looking set of wheels! The green eyed tint on Jenn's face only deepened just as the bus conductor popped up behind us asked for her email address…

*   *   *

Part Two – The Date!

A hotly anticipated affair. Since we'd already got the potentially awkward first meeting out of the way by meeting at the singles night, I was looking forward to seeing Karl again in a more private setting.

As I set off, I sent him a quick text to say I was on my way and whizzed off to meet him for lunch. The pub we'd chosen to eat at was in a pretty village, looking even better for the lovely weather we had that day (how typically English do I sound right now?).

I'd beaten Karl to the picnic table meeting point, so I ordered a drink and basked in the sunshine. I don't mind being the first there. It's nice to be able to relax before the date arrives anyway. However, after 10 minutes of waiting for Karl, I called him 10 minutes is a good rule I think, not appearing too panicked or paranoid – it's definitely worth checking to see if they're lost. However, he didn't pick up so after another five minutes of waiting, I went home with my tail between my legs.

When I got home I logged onto the dating site and I saw his profile said Karl had been online to check his email one minute before we were due to meet. Caught him! He'd obviously had no intention of meeting me for lunch. I sent him a snotty email and enjoyed doing so. He said he was ill, but I thought he could have picked up my call or text me at least. Oh well. If he was serious about meeting up, he'd call again… and he didn't.

What is with time wasters? Fair enough if they change their mind - I'm not naïve enough to think people don't chicken out, nor am I big-headed enough to think that I'm everyone's cup of tea, (and neither is online dating for that fact), but hey, give me a head's up before I take time out of my day to meet you for nothing. So much for the singles' night!

StarWars_Seth

29 years old

6'0'' tall, slim build

Milton Keynes

Describe yourself…

I'm Milton Keynes born and bred, and I'm looking for something a little more serious than my previous experience has provided in the dating department. A bit about me… I love films like the Bond films, Mission Impossible, Crank, (well, any action films really), and of course, Star Wars. I try to live life for the moment - this is the first time I've searched online for a date, (honest!!), not sure what to expect!

What are you looking for?

I'm looking for someone who's different from the rest, who can make me laugh and who doesn't mind me shouting at the rugby every other week! I love women with big smiles and friendly personalities, who aren't afraid to seize the day.

A Superhero?

Star Wars fan Seth was another online date that same summer. We had been talking for the obligatory couple of weeks online and, again, he seemed to be a nice guy. Apart from his interests in everything galactic, he ticked the intelligence box, and we seemed to have a few things in common – dog fans and a keen interest in action movies was a good start. More to the point, he lived round the corner from me. How convenient! I hoped we'd get along – if not, it could be awkward should we bump into each other in the street!

So, when the annual Milton Keynes geek fantasy convention came around and I heard some cast members from my favourite show 'Heroes' were going to be there, I thought what the heck, I'll invite Seth out for the day. The website promised an appearance from the droids for the Star Wars fans, so he'd probably enjoy the Star Wars. Together we could fight off any imposing Trekkies.

We met at the shopping centre and I quickly realised things weren't going to work out romantically - we just had no spark. There's got to be something exciting between you for sure. He was pretty quiet too, so it was hard work getting him to open up and relax. We supped our coffees and, yes, I was right - he was a nice enough guy. There was just one problem – there wasn't much attraction from my perspective. Who knows, maybe he felt the same way about me? He'd been single for over three years, so maybe he was the picky sort.

Seth did impart a piece of dating wisdom on me though when we were discussing our online experiences so far. An app is now available for iPhones which use a GPS tracking system to locate nearby potential dates (single people registered on the website). The app highlights people who have a similar type of music taste, according to which tunes you have stored on your iPhone. It sounded promising – we all know music is a good ice breaker! Too bad I don't have an iPhone… Seth didn't seem to have had much success with it though, since he was on a non-iPhone app date with me that morning. Maybe he had some embarrassing tracks on his phone that no one could relate to. The Smurfs Christmas CD, anyone?

After coffee, we wandered round the Comic-on style exhibits. Only one of the 'Heroes' characters showed up which was disappointing (and he was a rubbish one who only made an appearance in a couple of episodes), but Seth and I had our pictures taken with some Storm Troopers and had a giggle at the professional geeks wandering around. Fair dues to them, I guess - where else would you wear you Star Trek outfit if not to a geek convention?

When we parted company, Seth told me he'd like to see me again. I told Seth I'd really rather be friends and he consequently ignored my friendly "thanks for a nice day" email. Men are rubbish at being rude. I suppose ignoring someone is simply easier. Let's just hope we don't run into each other since we live near each other. Incidentally, I've noticed the convention looks even more ropey and extremely geeky this year. Best avoided maybe.

What are the rules of a threesome?

One night in March last year, Housemate Tom and I were out on the town, having a great time boogying on the dance floor of our favourite retro haunt, and getting very merry. I started talking to two guys, Martin and Jack from Milton Keynes, while Tom was at the bar. I decided surprisingly quickly that I'd be happy with either of them giving me their numbers – what an old trollop I am. It was probably all the vodka. So, while each one took turns to buy drinks, all three of us danced and they each chatted me up.

They worked out over the next hour or so that I wasn't a push over, and Jack pointed out I had more smarts than the typical bar fly he'd met, and seemed like I had a decent brain between my ears.

At the end of the night, Martin gave me his number, and offered an after party of sorts back at his place, with Jack. I politely declined, not wanting to get into some dodgy threesome with some guys I'd just met, and said "I'm here with my housemate, we're off home".

"Husband?" Martin shrugged. "Fine by us, bring him along too. Did I not say? We're married as well!"

I almost wet myself on the spot laughing at the fact that the loud music and my slurred speech rendered me married according to these guys, and that they were trying to entice me into a married couples' orgy. I left them waving their phones at me and went off to hail a cab with my housemate. Not husband. For all my smarts, I can still be a little embarrassingly naïve, but maybe now I know a little more.

Whatever the rules of threesome are of a giant orgy of apparently married people, I think I did it wrong. I did manage to escape before it was too late with my dignity still in tact though. I would be too much of a 'participant' to let someone else hog all the fun all night right in front of me. Sharing is not something I want in a relationship, unless it's regarding splitting the driving or the chores.

River_Rider

28 years old

5'8'' tall, average build

Milton Keynes

Describe yourself…

I'm an adventure seeker, my main passion is white water rafting and canoeing. If you've never tried rafting at the Aquadrome in Northampton I'd be happy to show you the ropes. I also enjoy snow boarding and mountain biking – if you think you can keep up, apply here!

What are you looking for?

We've got to be able to have a laugh and share similar tastes and conversation. I'm here to find a girlfriend, not a "flash in the pan" event…!

River Rider – Rock my boat?

Ever heard of 'Six Degrees of Separation'? It's the theory that you only need to know one person, who knows another, repeat to include three more people in the equation, and you can connect everyone in the world through normal everyday relationships and acquaintances. It turned out 'River Rider', also known as Connor, knew several people I did, having both worked for local Councils. Coincidental, but nice familiar territory, as I'm not from round here. Local Authorities do tend to move in small circles. It gave us a good ice breaking common ground to natter about, and let me see further than his Ted Baker suit.

We'd both admitted to having been on a few online dates before, so I tried to initiate a light-hearted discussion about the characters we'd met in the last few months, but Connor wasn't keen to share any gems. I guess some guys can get a bit precious about unsuccessful romantic encounters with women.

Connor had recently branched out away from normal internet dating websites and logged on to a dating website for bookworms. I forget its name, but you essentially list books you've enjoyed and the website recommends other single bookworms for you to get in touch with. Sounds interesting, a little like superhero Seth's iPhone app but for book-lovers, but I don't think I'd like to label myself by the books I read. I read crime, travel, biography, romance, adventure - even the occasional erotica. I like to think I am too varied in my reading to be pigeon-holed like that, but who knows, it might work for some.

Connor was as ruggedly handsome as they come, friendly, confident, appeared to be quite well-off, but he drove a huge penis extension of a car. Yes, a nice car is, well, nice, but money doesn't entertain me. Was Connor trying to impress me? Money talks, but it's a boring conversation. If he wanted a materialistic gold digger he was talking to the wrong woman. Funny how you can talk to someone for weeks, meet with them, and then cut all contact altogether, for ever. It's not how social situations normally work, but I supposed online dating isn't that 'normal'. Feelings probably mutual, we just went home after a couple of drinks and didn't bother contacting each other again. Easy!

Athleticism

Beardy Bedford

Beardy Bedford was a more run-of-the-mill non-online meeting. He was a footballer I met in a night club in Milton Keynes, but I think he's worth mentioning as it's an amusing story. Beardy Bedford was named that as he had a beard, he was from Bedford, and I still can't remember his actual name.

Isn't it odd how stepping into a nightclub erases social norms. Anywhere else, being approached by a stranger is an imposition. Where else would a stranger pinch your arse? Where else could it be possible to snog someone within two minutes of meeting them? Where else would the fail safe nightclub pickup lines like "hi gorgeous" or "come over here, love" work? I wonder when it becomes ok to even compliment a stranger on the street, let alone jump down to visit their tonsils. This behaviour is limited to a night club scene, and rightly so! Once you step through the gates of the cattle market that is Oceana, Milton Keynes, anyone is fair game it seems! In my eyes, chivalry beats a wolf-whistle or a compliment directed to my chest, based a little less on a Neanderthal's flirt tactics. We all know men don't always think with their brains, but it doesn't take many brains to be polite.

Beardy wasn't so primitive, despite his wholesome beard (mmm, rugged!). He was a confident guy, offering to buy me a drink and actually bothering to talk to me, as much as you can over the DJ. Ultimately we did end up joined at the lips. Now I'm never one to deny pleasure in a 'pull' when out for the night, but there's always risks when engaging with strangers. You never know how the smooch will work out, how they're going to react, even if you've spent most of the night chatting.

We exchanged numbers and made plans to meet up the next weekend for lunch in Oxford. I thought that was a bit far out the way for someone from Bedford, but whatever. I was more than happy to go to Oxford for the afternoon. I was already making mental notes as to where we should eat and drink, being a regular tourist to that part of the world.

It turns out Beardy was visiting a friend who lived in Bedford that night, and he was actually from Portsmouth. We decided we lived a little too far from each other, so we called it all off. I sure he wouldn't have *ran* all the way from Portsmouth to Milton Keynes just to take me out to dinner, as athletic as he was!

Sloppy Seconds don't work!

Simon was a guy my friend set me up with, hence the absence of the online profile page like most of my dates in this book. Jenn, over ten years older than Simon, thought the age gap between the two of them was too great, and recommended I took over the reigns. Here's a question – how many of your guy friends (previous love interest or not) would you recommend to a friend on the prowl? Not many, I'd hazard a guess. I am struggling to count beyond three fingers right now for example from my (few) close single guy friends. I wonder how serious Jenn was about me taking Simon for a test drive.

I wasn't convinced Simon was up for being passed about like a hot potato (albeit a very hot potato) but he called me the same evening Jenn had given him my phone number. He sounded very nice, and he wanted to call me again at the weekend as he was busy with work that week. Then maybe, he suggested, we could make some plans?

Anyway, after the weekend, I realised Simon only wanted me in his Little Black Book for when he came down to Buckinghamshire on a hockey tour. He was a goal tender for his local team – did I forget to mention? Mmm that would have been nice… But, to cancel that out, all Simon talked about was how busy he was and how boring his job was. If you don't like it, change it! Who's next?

Looking4Love

26 years old

5'8'' tall, average build

Northampton

Describe yourself…

I'm adventurous – my next challenge is a canyon swing I've booked for my holiday in New Zealand this Spring. I've got a big friendly chocolate Lab who had puppies last year – they didn't take long to find owners for, they were beautiful! I had training in Karate when I was a kid and recently have started training again, as well as going to the gym several times a week. I really enjoy it, and it gives me a good work out. And in case you're wondering, just because I keep myself trim it doesn't mean I'm a brainless idiot!

What are you looking for?

I'm only on here for genuine reasons, so jokers need not apply! ☺

Skint Steve

Skint Steve. There's not much to say about this encounter, and you can probably guess the content of this scenario from the title. Steve did sound like a winner from his profile. A picture perfect male. He was a dog lover, a perfect age and height for me, a keen traveller, and, of course, a strong interest in a sport ticks my 'athleticism' box! Nothing to fault there – let's see how this goes.

Steve was a little keen on making a date for our first meeting. That normally puts me off, but with so much going for him on his profile, I thought why not, we'd surely have loads to talk about. I'd actually been to New Zealand recently myself (see chapter on 'curious interest in the world'), so maybe I could suggest places to visit on his forthcoming trip, if nothing else cropped up in conversation. Things were looking up, finally!

After two weeks playing it cool, I agreed to a date with Steve. The evening before we were due to meet, Steve emailed me to ask if he could borrow £20 for the occasion. He said he wanted to be 'a gentleman' and pay for the drinks all night, but he was penniless. What a gentleman, scrounging off me before we'd even met. And a twenty for a night out? You need more than that! Hey, you know, just let me worry about the money, honey!

Any 'gents' who might be reading this, I'd think this was an obvious observation, but most girls won't want to subsidise their date from the word go, even if they're into equality of the sexes. Asking for a loan on the first date? No thanks, Steve. He was the athlete with a curious interest in the world, the date who ticked a lot of boxes, but the one I never met.

Back in the Computer Repair Shop

When that week with the particularly uneventful dates with Skint Steve and the joint disasters of Beardy Bedford and Sloppy Seconds Simon had ended, I couldn't resist it. Something pulled me back to the computer shop the first opportunity I had Monday morning. Perhaps it was primitive call of a certain tanned bod I knew would be chilling out, quietly working his computer fixing magic. I certainly didn't have any more problems with my laptop. It was working better than ever, thanks to Max. I'd have to pretend to be in urgent need of some blank CDs or something.

The shop was empty, even behind the counter. Mondays must be a quiet day in computer repairs. Perhaps people haven't had time in the week yet to mess them all up! I closed the glass paned door perhaps a little too hard to announce my arrival to Max, who was probably pottering about in the back somewhere.

"Hello?" I called.

"Hello there!" came the deep reply. Too deep. That wasn't Max. "I'll be out in a sec." That voice was definitely not Max. I hesitated. Was it too late to make a hasty exit?

"Is Max around?"

A tubby middle aged man emerging from the back of the shop. "Sorry love, he's got a day off today – Mondays are football training nights I believe. I can't keep up with that social butterfly."

Disappointed I'd missed out on seeing Max that morning, I caught myself wondering what else he got up to in his free time. Here was another footballer. That gave me a funny, familiar feeling inside.

On the spot, I caved in. "Ah, no problem. I was only after a couple of CDs really." A lucky sale for the shop. I couldn't just stand there and stare at the fat manager behind the counter. Maybe they should give Max more days off to boost their small item sales.

Hurrying out of the shop, clutching my new blank discs, I didn't think I'd be back again any time soon. For one thing, that was too embarrassing, and I couldn't think of a name of anything else I'd need for my computer. Wires and cables baffle me. Were those little storage things called Pin Sticks? 'UBS' thingys? I don't know… I'd feel silly going in again on a ruse of buying something else. I quit skiving work and made my way back to the office, a little disheartened. Max would have been sure to brighten my Monday morning, but obviously it was not to be.

Ambrose, my Taylor Swift date would have fitted nicely into this check-box, since our first date was to a music concert. However, his family still would have been in attendance and loads of potential dates have great taste in music and films, so there must be a man with similar interests to me who shares that all-important 'frisson' with me. Somewhere?

Craig, from 'The Toon'

It was a Sunday evening. Not wanting the weekend to end just yet, I had the impulse to go out on the town. My housemate Tom and I decided we could still get away with it on a 'school night' – especially Tom, who, lucky bugger, had no work the next morning.

By 9.30pm we were stationed at a table in Lloyd's Bar, which became the only prop Tom would have to hold himself up with by the end of the night. I was driving, for simplicity (it wasn't going to be complicated getting a wasted housemate home with me in a few hours), so I wasn't drinking. Tom started chucking drinks down his throat, and wouldn't dance, so I took to the near-by dance floor by myself. Almost every other song was a karaoke track, but before long I was surrounded by men, so I wasn't short of a dance partner. I was in my own little world, laughing and dancing away to a few men attempting to impersonate Take That (love that song!). One of them just happened to be quite good looking. That was Craig.

While we were dancing, we chatted a little. He said was 22 years old (a toy boy!), and from 'The Toon'. Over the loud music and my southern England ignorance of most things north of Birmingham, I thought he meant he was from 'the town', (i.e. Milton Keynes centre). Later that week Housemate Tom would confirm my suspicions that I didn't think Craig was in it for the long-term by enlightening me on the facts that 'The Toon' was slang for Newcastle, not 'the town'. What a numpty I was. Craig certainly didn't fit my 'living close by' criteria then!

Anyway, back to that Sunday night. I had a few drinks with Craig and his friends at the bar, glancing to check on Tom who was getting more and more wasted in the corner, eyeing up two women, obviously lesbians, sitting at the next table. It wasn't long before he was so drunk he couldn't sit on his chair, so come midnight we went home. Craig and I had exchanged numbers but I didn't expect to see him again. It was just a really fun night out, and I never felt better on a Monday morning than I did that week.

Craig called that evening and we made plans to go out for drinks on the Tuesday. We had a few drinks in Revolution bar in town, and then got a takeaway on the way home. Dates at my house are normally not on the cards for a couple of weeks, but I knew it was my pad, my rules. I can bend them when and where I like, thank you!

Craig was working as a carpenter who was helping to renovate a nightclub in Milton Keynes for the next three weeks. He had nothing to do in the evenings while living in a temporary apartment. He shared it with a painter colleague who wasn't much fun, so I became his local entertainment and we went out several nights in the next few weeks.

Date three was a meal out in Nando's chicken place. I've not been blown away by Nando's before, (see Albanian Arben's chapter), but Craig said he'd never tried it, so that was our eatery for that evening. I can't remember what I ordered, but Craig had nachos with chilli, sour cream and guacamole.

When the meal arrived, Craig pointed at the guacamole, (incidentally, one of my favourite dips), and said "what's that green lumpy shit?"

Ok, so it's not that common a dish, but it's not unusual, especially when served with nachos. It was on the menu's description of the nacho main, so I thought it a bit weird that he wasn't expecting to see guacamole on his plate.

"It's a kind of dip made of vinegar, mayonnaise, avocado etc," I replied gently.

"What's avocado?" he replied.

Oh wow, what a match we were. He didn't even know what an avocado is, one of my favourite foods. Worrying times – I can't date someone who's not adventurous about food, and annoyingly fussy about it too. I just can't. I'll eat anything. Fish balls? Done. Kangaroo and ostrich steaks? Done. I have yet to level with my Dad's adventurous appetite (he's tried bull's balls), but I am proud of having enjoyed frogs legs and snails in the past.

Anyway, we managed to gloss over his fussiness and ignorant cuisine tastes, and we spent the rest of the evening in the nightclub he was renovating during the daylight hours. We got free

VIP access and drinks all night – possibly why most of our dates involved heavy drinking and lots of dancing.

Despite his cuisine caution, things were going well. He was lots of fun, good looking, and was into the same music as me. He was polite and easy going, and despite a good portion of what he was saying was lost on me due to his thick Geordie accent, we got on really well.

The last night he was in Milton Keynes, I brought him home for the night. We continued to have a good night there too, if you catch my drift…But he couldn't get my bra off. Any man who can't even unfasten a bra, with the lights on, when they're looking so closely at the catch they're scrutinising my skin cells does not deserve the goods if you ask me. Hopefully attempting to take my bra off was a move of foreplay and he didn't want to try it on for himself. Been there, seen that, biggest turn-off ever. But I'll never know. Unfortunately for my dwindling sex life, we didn't get much further, and fell into a drunken stupor.

Craig went back to Newcastle that weekend and we've since lost touch. I hope he's doing alright back 'oop norf'. He was a nice guy, but there was no chance we were going to be able to make a relationship work over a distance of 230 miles. Long distance ain't my bag, baby! There's no amount of music and films to keep me occupied on *that* train journey.

The Tourist

Scene set: I was enjoying my final night out on a 16 day trip visiting some girl friends in Canada. It was 'Freshers' Week' at the university they all studied at, so you can imagine what a raucous couple of weeks they were. A couple of us ended up in a local haunt called 'Big Bucks' this particular evening, a favourite haunt of mine as it was decked out as a hunting lodge. I've never seen one like that in the UK, that's for sure.

My friend Maddy and I got to dancing, drinking, and eyeing up the rugged scenery surrounding us (and I don't mean taxidermist's triumphs hanging from the wall!). I started talking to a guy named Braydon outside on the smoking terrace when I was out getting some fresh air. I know, 'fresh' air on a smoking terrace doesn't really happen, but it was better that than the probable consequences of me not clearing my head with some summer evening breeze after that many cocktails.

I can't remember what we talked about posing on the balcony, and couldn't remember in morning either, but Maddy said he gave us his cab home and the email address I found scrawled on the shirt sleeves I'd worn out that night was his. 'WhiteWizard2000'. I laughed – what saddo has a Lord of the Rings reference in his email? I thought nothing more of it and assumed I'd not hear from him again, let alone see him. I flew back to the UK and slept off my multiple hangovers and jet lag from a long trip home.

When I arrived back home in my student digs, there was an email waiting for me in my inbox. You've got mail! And you can guess who it was from – it turns out I gave Braydon my email too that night. It was a nice message, hoping I'd had a safe journey home, and telling me he'd quit cigarettes since meeting me. On my request apparently!

Of course, I replied. We'd had a great time and he'd been nice to check I got home ok. Our emails developed into an on-and-off four week chat via email/MSN chat/webcams between my classes, social life, studying and the rest of what university life brings.

He was 29 to my younger 21, he was tall at 6'6" (I remembered that much from our night out!), and I learnt a lot about the town he lived in. I knew about his job as a Sheraton hotel employee, learnt about his dreams, ambitions and his family problems. We also shared the same passion for country music and meeting new people. I was filled in on what he loves to do with his time (namely following the band Blue Rodeo around the country), and, strangely, how he'd never left the country. He didn't even own a passport! That concept was totally alien to me. I can't sit still, always exploring and finding somewhere new to visit. How would I ever have met Braydon for instance, 3,000 miles away, without a passport?

Due to the time difference, Braydon would be waking up just as I'd be coming home for lunch so we had a lot of lunch/breakfast dates before he headed off to work. When he came home from work I could be on my way to bed, so we were a bit out of synch, but over those few weeks I got to know him intrinsically. So well in fact that when he said he'd organised a passport and bought tickets to come visit me, I couldn't hide my excitement.

Braydon visited for five nights during my October reading week in which I did no reading. We went out on the town every night and took a weekend trip to London to see the sights. Ever the tourist, I had a great time showing him the fantastic locations in London, including Big Ben, ("hilarious name for a clock!"), stealing some pebbles from Buckingham Palace's driveway ("Bucking-HAM Palace" in his endearing accent), and the numerous museums. We even managed to squeeze in some sights which were slightly off the beaten track. We were both fans of The Ashes cricket series, so I took him to Lord's ground, and I was probably more than a little more excited than him when we hunted down the house the Channel 4 series 'Spaced' was filmed at. I'd managed to get Braydon hooked on the show in the few days he was visiting, so that was a private triumph for us, seeking out that hidden house in North London.

Braydon was excellent fun. We were always laughing and larking about, flirting and chatting. Come to think of it, he was probably constantly tipsy, which would have helped. Can you blame the guy? He was on 'vacation' after all! Still, we had a fantastically enjoyable time in London and I was sad to see him leave for the airport on Monday morning.

* * *

Four months passed, and our online 'meets' became fewer and shorter. After all, I had a life away from the computer and a degree to complete. However, at the end of January, Braydon announced he'd gotten a tattoo to commemorate his first trip abroad to see me and our shared interest in The Ashes season. He'd bought a plane ticket to come and see me again, the weekend after my birthday, keen to show off his new body artwork. I'm not a big fan of tattoos and his description didn't sound amazing... In addition to this, his second trip was more out-of-the-blue and unexpected than the first time as I felt we were kind of growing away from each other. That was normal, I imagined, since we lived so far apart and no real relationship could be sustained via webcam anyway, surely!? He didn't seem to think the same as me though. He was virtually packed and ready to go. What could I say?!

So Braydon arrived on the train from Heathrow, grinning excitedly and clutching some ugly blue roses. Horrible! Roses should only ever be white, pink or red in my opinion. He was in a hurry to dump his bags on the platform and quickly rolled up his sleeve to show me his tattoo. He was so proud of it but it was dreadful. There were way too many colours in the design, and he'd made an awful pun of the word 'cricket' inferring to the game, by designing an actual insect cricket on top of a cricket bat. To top it off, the cricket bat, normally a beautiful creamy colour carved in willow wood, was plastered in the Union Jack. Our long weekend had not started well.

Braydon came to stay for just three nights that February due to work pressures. We had a nice enough time, but any budding or potential romance had long since dissipated. It felt more than a little awkward at times, and I think he expected more. A night away in Chester in a luxurious and decadent hotel room (a Sheraton employee benefit rate of course!) did nothing to tempt me into his aching arms. Apart from anything else, I didn't want to see anymore badly designed tattoos which he may have had. I'd long since reclassified him in my head away from boyfriend material and into a 'friend' category – this relationship was never going to bloom over the distance of 'The Pond'. And when I tactfully explained this to him, he walked out, bummed a cigarette off a neighbour, and stole my suitcase. My favourite Quiksilver holdall. I still haven't forgiven him for that! I never saw or heard from him (or the suitcase!) again.

I feel a little bit guilty about the whole situation really, perhaps having maybe led him on a little, but how could I stop him buying a plane ticket to come and see me?! I was still young, naïve even, but I learnt a lot from this gem. Most people don't see the world, their relationships, obstacles and reasoning the same way as you might.

Lunch Time Loving

I met Jeremy about half way through my year working in Canada, the same year I met Toronto Joe of the Toblerone cake fame. Jeremy wanted a job as an Air Quality Tester, like I had. Lucky me, I was nominated as his trainer. It was a good temporary job for someone like me on a limited visa, but perhaps not a great career move for a home-grown Canadian with half a brain. He was cute, he had a bright smile, and he played the drums. I don't seem to come across many musical blokes - I was secretly pleased I was ranking Air Quality Tester for the day when I was assigned the new trainee to show him the ropes.

So, I don't know how much you know about air quality or the testing of it, and I won't bore you, but our job essentially involved collecting a sample of air from pre-booked appointments at people's homes and taking the 10 or so samples we collected each day back to the lab. It used a lot of petrol, but the bosses were fair enough and the social scene within the team was great. We had a couple of office parties every week and I felt very well included and looked after for a young girl on foreign turf. I could count on these guys and we became quite like a little family with my 'older brothers' looking out for me.

Jeremy was a welcome new addition to the group, the guys at work approved clearly, and we happily spent the training day together cooped up in my car cruising around to appointments. We laughed at the oddballs we called on, and played DJ with the new iPod I'd bought the previous weekend. Jeremy took great pleasure at showing his disgust at my country music playlist, but I caught him singing along more than once. You can't help but know the words when you live in a country like Canada, the music is everywhere. We even had a CD swapping session when I dropped him home (including some country classics!). He was quiet, but Jeremy loosened up soon enough. Quite a bit by the end actually. By noon we were 'pashing' (as they say in Canada) in the driver's seat, and it more than made my day. That day's lunch break was the best I've enjoyed – ever!

Once Jeremy was fully trained up, he was off on his own in the exciting world of air quality testing, and we started seeing a bit of each other out of work. We were the 'work couple' at the next office keg party, we spent a couple of evenings in his flat watching DVDs – he had a great selection I hadn't seen before – and we went out for dinner once or twice. I even got a few drum lessons thrown in for good measure. Jeremy was still pretty quiet, but he was too easy on the eyes to worry. I have no problem filling silences myself anyway. However, after two weeks of this, it did get a little tedious.

I can't tell you much more about Jeremy as he didn't speak up a lot. The last time I saw him was the final time because he piped up with the unforgettable line "I just like listening to you talking in your British accent". Not music to my ears, I can tell you!

Jeremy quit the air testing company soon afterwards. I think he was another example of a North American after some fresh foreign fish. Perhaps he should search for his green card, sorry, his soul mate on a website like www.iloveyouraccent.com.

ASH_2006

26 years old

6' tall, average build

Northampton

Describe yourself…

Tall, dark, fun-loving, confident guy, who's sick of seeing the normal UK tourist sights. I want to see the world!!! I am planning a fortnight in The Gambia this December, but I'd love to meet someone who shares my wander lust. I enjoy playing tennis and football, supporting my local team in Northampton.

What are you looking for?

I'm looking for something long-term, not a "quick-fix".

The Day I Was Bored – Part One

Ashley was boredom killer date number one. Navy Nathan followed for date two that day, but we'll get to him in due course.

Ashley and I went to see new Simpsons movie at the cinema. We went to the bar upstairs at Cineworld beforehand to chat and get to know each other a bit, but I really rather wish we hadn't bothered at all. Hindsight is always 20:20, a wise friend of mine always says.

Cinema dates – pros and cons…

X   It's dark in the theatre which makes it hard to perve on your hot date, and the arm rests limit your movements towards affection

√   It's dark in the theatre which makes it hard to perve on your hot date, and the arm rests limit your movements towards affection (yes, intended repetition here!)

√   You get to see a film, and if he's a gent, he'll let you choose

X   Not much opportunity to get chatting without being thrown out

√   Popcorn – 'nuff said, lovely stuff!

X   Cinema's not the cheapest option nowadays. Prices never fail to surprise me in theatres nowadays.

Ashley was 15 minutes late (what is it with guys being late?!), and when he came to the top of the stairs I almost didn't recognise him. Instead of the 'tall dark haired' man I was expecting from the information on his profile, he was well under the promised six foot tall, and he had ginger hair.

This guy's first sentence involved a nasty comment about his ex-girlfriend – what a first date taboo. I'm not interested in her. I already know I will never be her. I'm no one's rebound sounding board. Added to that, Ashley appeared to despise his family (not an attractive trait) and, I'm not a prudish person, but he made some pretty inappropriate comments about the goodies on the nearby hotdog stand.

There was a third seat at our table and a woman loitering near-by asked us if she could use it. *'Please, come join us,'* I thought. *'Take my seat, you're welcome to it!'* I jumped at the chance of different conversation and she accepted my heartfelt invitation to sit with us until her own date arrived. She joined us for almost 20 minutes. They were the most enjoyable 20 minutes of the night.

Ashley, I and a couple of tumbleweeds finally moved off to the cinema screen, via a quick trip to the Ladies for me. I sent a text message to my friend Jenn from there, cowering by the sinks.

Just a quick message, I swear, laughing that I already had a brilliantly awful dating story to tell her.

I apparently took so long in the loos that Ashley found it apt to ask me outright when I rejoined him in the hallway if I had a bladder problem. What the hell was he thinking? Tempting as it was to run off, I was still looking forward to the greatly anticipated Simpsons screening, and the 'no talking' rule in the theatre was going to be an added bonus. At this point, I'd stopped pretending to myself we would have something, somewhere, in common. Yes, we both enjoyed the same sort of films, but I was not going to search deeper for something more poetic or profound.

The film was brilliant, I definitely recommend it, but I don't recommend taking Ashley along with you. The film wasn't in anyway romantic being a feature length Simpsons episode, (thank God), but somehow the cheesy old trick of the man stretching and reaching round his unsuspecting date's shoulders was too tempting to resist for Ashley. I squirmed into the far corner of my seat, making it *quite* clear I wanted no funny business from him, thank you. Yuck! Lord only knows how I made it through the film.

After the film, I hurried my coat on and sharply marched it out of the cinema. Ashley ran after me in the rain shouting that we should go and see another film next weekend, so I called back "text me!" knowing full well he didn't have my number. Yeah, you do that. Text me.

Mean? Not at all - necessary! Navy Nathan, part two of my fun-filled day, can be found in the next chapter. The criteria? Uniforms!!!

NavyNathan08

22 years old

5'7'' tall, average build

Northampton

Describe yourself…

Hi – my name's Nathan and I'm in the Navy. I am home for 6 months and looking to meet someone I can come home to when I'm on leave, especially since it's almost Christmas!

I'm into personal fitness, chart music, and I love tower running, brown sauce & ketchup – I don't know what I'd do without my "rescue rations" condiments on board ship!

What are you looking for?

See above – I'm particularly partial to brunettes, so if you'd like to meet a real man, apply here!

The Day I Was Bored – Part Two

I learned a lot from today. I recovered from Ashley and the Simpson movie debacle and went to dinner with Navy Nathan. I am not going to do two dates in one day just because I'm bored again. Ever. I find that if I'm not particularly looking forward to meeting a bloke, I find I'm not that keen or enthusiastic about the dates at all. Gut feelings are a good thing to pay attention to – I should know that by now. These two dates were probably at the peak of my serial online dating habit…

The second guy on that boring Sunday was a sailor, home from the Navy, as you can see from his profile. Boredom should not be taken so lightly. I left my house already knowing this wouldn't work. I was more than deflated from the cinema trip with Ashley, and I can't imagine having my man the other side of the world for months at a time, potentially involved in armed conflict, as it could one day be with Nathan.

Dinner – pros and cons…

√   You get fed (obviously!) – everyone loves a fresh summer restaurant menu

X   Public embarrassment of being stood up if the worst happens. Not good!

√   No lack of conversation – the venue, the food/drink, even the other customers if you get *that* bored

X   Lost in translation – make sure you know what you're ordering. No one wants an allergic reaction when you've ordered snails (escargots) thinking it was a turkey escalope

√   Dinner can be as long (or short) as you wish it to be. If it's floundering in the shallows, you can decline pudding or turn down the coffee afterwards.

X   The awkward moment of paying the bill. Do you act old fashioned and let him pay? Do you go Dutch and split it equally? On the first date I offer to halve it, as I reckon if he's not enjoyed the date (more fool him but) he shouldn't have to pay it all. I'm not a bra-burning feminist, but I am a modern woman.

Nathan was full of drunken Naval stories that I don't have a lot to relate to with, but at least it was different to the normally conversations I've had. Still, he virtually left the restaurant to return to his submarine, and I left the restaurant thinking that maybe it was marginally better as the date with Ashley earlier. Anything would be an improvement on that one, but Nathan firmly cemented my views that a military man is not for me.

Chinese Charlie

This is a genuine 'out of the blue' email I received from Charlie, a Chinese guy living in Peterborough. Apparently the dating website we both belonged to thought we were a compatible match so they allegedly recommended that he should send me an email. I have obviously made his details anonymous but you still get the idea of his literary and romantic genius…

---

hiya,
its doesnt matter, matched just our mutual friend, its a tool, ok, let me be directly tellin you that i want a real gf, *(girlfriend)* i am very honest! i believe God! i am also a christion!
and ok,we can both leaving from the website, my membership till july, but its ok, u can have my mobile number, i am serious and my culture only allow me to marry once in my lifetime, then i value you! i try to find out a real gf who i can going to marry with,
then give me text msg*(message)*,
07*** ******
and my msn, i will online after 3pm,coz my work off late, i wish u can move to me, hehe, Peterborough, cambridgeshire,
Charlie**********@hotmail.com
wish to hear from you about good news that you want to developefuthure with me!
plz*(please)*!
yours Charlie!

He seems excited with all his !!! punctuation, and wants to 'value' me, but I found Charlie's email ridiculous, more than a little too keen. I also have a 'pet peev' of when people don't use proper language to write you a message. This might sound harsh as his first language obviously isn't English, but in general, if people "like 2 tlk like this I h8 communic8in wit em". It's ok to laugh obviously -

an occasional "lol" is fine – even if you're not actually Laughing Out Loud. In general though, 'netspeak' use normally ends in failure in my eyes.

Chinese Charlie did make an effort with his profile picture though – he looked like a naval officer of some kind. If you're in the armed forces, putting a picture up of you in uniform has *got* to help your cause in most cases. However, just knowing he wants me to move to Peterborough was enough reason to not reply. Anyone who knows about my bad experiences in that town would expect nothing less – I've had eventful visits up there before, having been chased by a beggar, not got a job I went to an interview for, and was once attacked by a blind man and his stick.

What did I learn from this one? Not a lot if, I am honest, but he was too hard to omit from this singleton's story. Bless him, Chinese Charlie had no chance. Next!

Curly_Chris

24 years old

5'8" tall, athletic build

Milton Keynes

Describe yourself…

I'm Chris, pleased to meet you. First of all thanks for looking at my profile – I'm not sure what to write to be honest! I'm a friendly, optimistic, sometimes a shy kind of guy, who'd like someone to share the fast-approaching winter evenings with. Everyone says you should try online dating, so here I am! I've been a policeman for 5 years now, and I love it. I feel privileged to have a job I enjoy so much! I'm a bit of a joker - I love to make people laugh.

What are you looking for?

What are YOU looking for? Some people are just too vague on here!

"Yes, Officer!"

At this point in my search I'd moved on from a free online dating site, as I got offered a great deal for a couple of months on a cheap-ish subscription site. My thoughts were, if I'm having no luck on the free one, maybe the people on the subscription service were a bit more genuine and serious about finding someone for the longer term

Chris was more than charming on email. He also waited until a few messages had passed between us to mention anything positive about my physical features, which I took as a good sign. Anyone who mentions how 'fit' you are or how gorgeous you look in your profile picture in the first couple of messages are a little creepy in my view, a total turn-off. Sometimes people seem to think compliments will get them anywhere, a means to an end...

I was recovering from a cold the evening we met, but so was Chris, so if all else failed we could be 'cold-buddies' at the very least. And in my experience, policemen always have a wealth of funny and cheeky stories to keep their audience entertained. I couldn't help entertaining myself with the thought of him bringing his handcuffs with him on our date...

As both of us were hampered by sore throats, a trip to the cinema seemed a good idea. We easily settled on seeing Jim Carey's "Yes Man", a new film neither of us had seen yet. Chris was sure it would make us laugh through the fog of head colds, plus, and I quote, "we didn't have to strain our sore throats talking all night". Oh, you charmer! Wait, why not add the fact that there was no physical activity at the cinema to threaten to wear us into the ground to your list rationalising our date activity?

I enjoyed the film, but the popcorn was more entertaining than this self-proclaimed 'joker'. I am afraid that's all I remember from that evening. It must have been fun. Lesson learnt – being a policeman doesn't mean you're full of fun and games, (kinky or otherwise), despite what I'd previously thought!

Hello Sailor!

On a cruise holiday away with my family, my Dad and I went out for a boogie in a club after the rest of the family went off to bed. Boring, you might think, a night out with your dad. But no - Dad's the life and soul of the party, and Cotton Eyed Joe's famous track never fails to remind me of him swinging perfect strangers around the floor. It was a great night, but I wanted to stay later that he did. Rule No.1 for responsible Dads: don't leave your daughter alone in a club surrounded by sailors.

This one particular sailor and I had a great time, dancing the night away in the on-board nightclub and drinking posh drinks. At the end of the night, he took me to see the engine room of the ship. Very impressive, a slightly sketchy 'off limits' place to be hidden away in, all excitement. He played the old trick of pretending to me higher in command than he actually was, initially fooling me I was flirting with the third in command, but having a look in the ships brochure the next day his name was nowhere to be seen. I never saw him again, but the uniform sticks in my mind for sure. How many women in how many ports do you think he had…?

This_is_me_24

24 years old

5'7" tall, athletic build

Luton

Describe yourself…

I grew up around here so I have quite a good network of mates and family. I'm a little shy, but I can come out of my shell very easily in the right circumstances. I enjoy good conversation and hanging out with my friends. I play for my local rugby team, and I'm a fireman - but don't let that put you off!!!

What are you looking for?

Compatibility in interests is key for me. Anyone who enjoys the same things as me has a better chance I'd imagine as we'd have things in common to talk about. I like blondes or brunettes, I'm not picky in that area!

Silence Is Golden

Ricky, from Luton. Bless him. I was looking forward to this date more than most others. After all, he was a fireman, for goodness sake! Perhaps to my detriment, I'd built him up to be some sort of wonder-man in my head beforehand though.

Ricky hardly said a word the whole hour we were sat awkwardly in the Fox and Hounds pub. And when he did speak, his tone was so soporific, and added to the effect of mid-afternoon drinking, I feared I might even need a nap before the evening really got started. There was little to no conversation, let alone any chemistry. I imagine that playing sports brings out confidence in adults, having seen it in kids' martial arts training sessions. Not in Ricky's case! Water out of a stone springs to mind… He bought me a couple of double vodka and cokes though, so I had no problem filling the silence with words. I asked questions, replied with questions, helped him answer my questions, and even answered my own. I prompted and encouraged, but it was like flogging a dead horse.

One gem Ricky *did* let slip was that he was one of those guys that's just soooo nice, and he thinks girls don't like him because they all secretly love idiots. I think blokes like this should take some time to look closely at themselves in the mirror and being honest with themselves – is there another reason women don't reply to their messages? I would have thought a fireman would be a bit more switched on than this…

My efforts continued. I touched on deep subjects, and then went back to shallow again. We (let's be honest, I) talked about the weather, the new Jay-Z CD, and I even resorted to telling him he was only the second Ricky I'd ever met in my entire life. Fascinating stuff.

Desperate for some light relief and as those couple of double vodka and cokes had flown through my system, I escaped to the Ladies' for a couple of minutes. I think I had more of a conversation laughing with a woman in typical girlie 'toilet chat' style in there in two minutes than I had all evening so far with Ricky.

A sneaky piece of Dutch courage was in order. I might as well enjoy myself – Ricky obviously had no 'get up and go', no fire in his belly – lucky for a fireman I suppose. How boring though! A quick couple of sweet apple flavoured shots later and I was again psyching myself up to return to our table round the corner from the bar.

Almost toppling on my heels, moving way too fast for a light-weight drinker like me, I accidentally bumped into the bloke standing next to me, ordering a pint. He immediately and unnecessarily apologised. I took a closer look.

It was Max from the computer repair shop. He was wearing a cobbled together football kit, fresh from the pitch from the look of the mud stains on his knees and the empty water bottle in his hand. Oh my, it was Max. Fearing my beer (ok, vodka) goggles had gotten the better of me, I wobbled. Mentally and physically. I was sure it was him. The athlete look sure suited him – as did the three or four day beard growth he was sporting.

A rugged looking athlete? Something suddenly cleared in my vodka veiled mind. It clicked. He ticked all the boxes.

Max was:

1. Chatty, yet thoughtful – his conversation, customer service and politeness showed that.
2. Interested in the world – I'd previously learned he was off to Canada in a few months
3. Interested in his own things – I certainly was no footballer but I'd be happy to accept the benefits from dating one.
4. Family orientated – planning his mum's surprise party convinced me of that. It's a lot of effort planning such a 'do', so I could assume he loved spending time with his family.
5. Intelligent. Significantly more than me when it comes to computers, at least!
6. He was suddenly looking rather rugged – I was loving the new bearded look!
7. A local. Quick access to him checks off criteria number seven for me!
8. Of course, athletic. Just look at those footballer's calves!
9. Into films and music – well, who isn't to some degree?
10. Even in possession of a uniform… of sorts. The not-so-hot blue and orange computer shop outfit will do for now. Well, he can't be perfect!

What a turn up for the books! Max has been there all along, quietly hiding in the background. Suddenly my evening in the Fox and Hounds looked a whole lot brighter.

Before I could concoct anything intelligent to say to Max through my vodka mist, he rescued me.

"Louise! Sorry, I didn't see you there." Wow, that smile blew me away. "How's the laptop?"

If I rocked back on my heels and squinted, I could just about see Ricky, day dreaming out the window. Something (probably a combination of my libido, my heart and the limits to my patience with people who aren't great conversationalists) told me to forget him. Fair enough, maybe Ricky was shy, but how can he expect for me to feel a spark with him when he would just sit quietly supping his pint? Sure, he was hot, and the fireman's uniform would surely come in useful had we progressed much further, but Ricky was too much like hard work.

Pulling myself together, I struck a more controlled, ladylike pose in my wobbly heels. Max and I flew through conversation like old friends. His family party went well the other week, work was going well, and his team won the football game that evening.

"I didn't know you drank here", he said, his dark eyes brows arching.

"Not often…" I replied. It suddenly dawned on me. I'd been absent from my unsuspecting date for almost 20 minutes now. Ricky was still sitting by the window, waiting for me to return from my loo break with the drinks. I couldn't order more now and prolong the agony any further. Sitting over there with him, attempting to drag words out of the quietest date I'd ever encountered now seemed like the trial of the century. I wanted to stay chatting with Max.

The drink was really started to hit me, and I needed to nip the fireman fiasco in the bud before Ricky noticed me flirting outrageously with someone else at the bar. I reluctantly made my excuses to take my leave from Max, but not before Max offered me his phone number and invited me out for sushi next weekend. A confident guy with adventurous tastes in food too – I like it. Eat your avocado ignorant heart out, Craig from 'The Toon'! Max was improving by the minute. I couldn't wait for the weekend. Muchos excitement!

I pulled myself together and stopped by the table Ricky was perched at on the way out. I explained I had to leave as my housemate needed collecting from the train station. That old chestnut.

Ricky chose this final moment of our date to pipe up – should I be driving in my condition? Concern mixed with bad timing of sudden interest and conversation led me to walk out with a dismissive wave and the obligatory quick and polite 'thank you for a lovely evening'.

Of course I wasn't driving – I virtually ran down the street home, clutching the napkin with Max's number written on it with joy. I'd got more than I'd ever thought possible from my date with Ricky.

An Ending

So, there you have it. A collection of dating stories you'd probably rather didn't happen to you, but did, word for word, happen to me. I was tempted to finish my book with a fabricated grand finale (a kidnapping maybe?! You and I both now know it's more than a plausible scenario looking at my track record!), but I think that would destroy the whole idea of this being genuine account of a young woman's rocky search for love.

What would have been a great ending is if it had turned out I was writing this reflecting back, on something like my 25th wedding anniversary or something similar. In reality, I am in my mid-twenties, sat in a Milton Keynes cafe typing my final chapters, patiently waiting for Max (my boyfriend!). I deliberately arrived earlier than we'd planned to meet. I wanted to wrap this book up, tie up the loose ends.

Max and I have been together almost a year now. He's thinking of starting his own computer repair business (with a nicer uniform I hope!), we're in the process of booking a holiday to Corfu this summer. He's still playing football and I ensure I regularly take advantage of his deliciously trim footballer's body. Although it's not a perfect story fairy tale ending with white horses and crowns, things are going great. I might not have had the guts to finish this off if I'd have still been single so I need to run off some prints before the potential for 'something bad' to happen. Hopefully it won't though – I've never felt this good about a relationship before. I hate that phrase 'the one', but…

As an added bonus, it's been great that I've made a couple of friends through my online shenanigans (e.g. Toronto Joe and Irish Ambrose from the Taylor Swift date), and mine and Jenn's friendship has become all that stronger as we shared our trials and tribulations from the online game. Max, however, is by far the best thing to come out of this story of ruffians, misfits and criminals.

To all you singletons out there who might be reading this - it's not the end of the world not being attached. So many people stay in a relationship 'just because', so keep looking after Number One (you!). Make sure you're happy and you're getting what you want out of any relationship. It's useful to bear in mind that no man is perfect – you just need to find the one who's perfect enough. I hope these stories have made you feel better about any bad dates you may have had, and they reassure you that you're not alone.

What did the Fab Four have to say? All you need is love. At the end of the day, dating is a numbers game. There's a huge pool of people out there – well over 40 million people online alone. Remember, there's plenty more fish in the sea. Happy dating!